THE COMPLETE CORTISOL DETOX HANDBOOK

A PRACTICAL GUIDE & WORKBOOK FOR BALANCING HORMONES, REGULATING EMOTIONS, HEALING YOUR GUT, REDUCING INFLAMMATION AND MANAGING STRESS

SAGE O'REILLEY

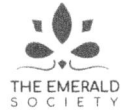

THE EMERALD SOCIETY

© **Copyright 2025 by The Emerald Society - All rights reserved.**

The content contained within this book may not be reproduced, duplicated, or transmitted without direct written permission from the author or the publisher.

Under no circumstances will any blame or legal responsibility be held against the publisher, or author, for any damages, reparation, or monetary loss due to the information contained within this book, either directly or indirectly.

Legal Notice:

This book is copyright protected. It is only for personal use. You cannot amend, distribute, sell, use, quote or paraphrase any part, or the content within this book, without the consent of the author or publisher.

Disclaimer Notice:

Please note that the information contained within this document is for educational and entertainment purposes only. All effort has been executed to present accurate, up-to-date, and reliable, complete information. No warranties of any kind are declared or implied. Readers acknowledge that the author is not engaging in the rendering of legal, financial, medical, or professional advice. The content within this book has been derived from various sources. Please consult a licensed professional before attempting any techniques outlined in this book.

By reading this document, the reader agrees that under no circumstances is the author responsible for any losses, direct or indirect, which are incurred as a result of the use of the information contained within this document, including but not limited to errors, omissions, or inaccuracies.

LEAVE A REVIEW

Don't forget to share the love and **leave your Amazon review** for:

The Complete Cortisol Detox Handbook

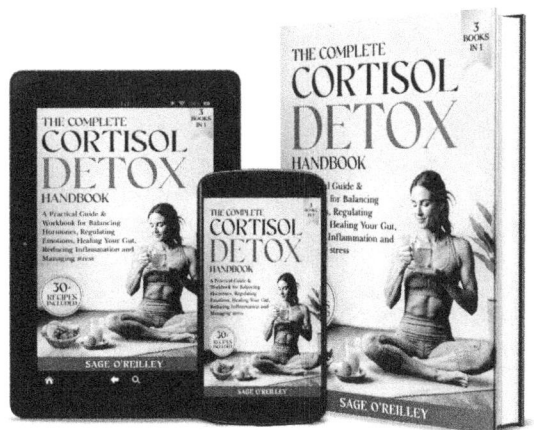

CONTENTS

Introduction	1
1. Understanding Cortisol and Its Impact	3
2. The Science of Detoxification	29
3. Nutrition for Hormonal Harmony	47
4. Exercise and Movement for Stress Reduction	63
5. Stress Management and Emotional Resilience	83
6. Lifestyle Changes for Long-Term Balance	104
7. Tackling the Hurdles of Cortisol Detox	116
Conclusion	128
BONUS: Top 30 Cortisol Detox Recipes	131
Postscript	156
Join Our Tribe	159
Bibliography	161

INTRODUCTION

IN THE QUIET moments of the night, when the world slows down and the noise fades, many women find themselves wide awake. Stress creeps in, casting shadows over their thoughts. It's a common story: juggling careers, family, and personal goals, all while feeling the weight of endless responsibilities. For many of us, stress transcends beyond a momentary emotion, becoming a relentless presence in our lives. Studies show that chronic stress affects nearly 75% of women, leading to a cascade of health issues. Unbeknown to us, at the heart of this storm is cortisol, playing havoc with our body and mind.

Cortisol imbalance goes beyond simple stress. It manifests as weight gain, mood swings, fatigue, and even disrupts our sleep. You may find yourself wondering why you're exhausted despite a full night's sleep or why those extra pounds won't budge. Well, within these pages, we will demystify the complex relationship between cortisol and its impact on our health. This is a tool developed to offer insights into how this protective hormone can contribute to weight gain, mood swings, fatigue, and sleep disturbances. Through a deeper understanding, we will uncover why, despite seemingly adequate rest, exhaustion still looms large, and why those stubborn pounds resist our best efforts to shed them.

So, together, let's peel back the layers of confusion surrounding cortisol and its influence on our health. Soon, you will have gained enough knowledge to design a clear plan to hack your hormones and live your best life. You'll also discover how to manage cortisol and improve your health through practical exercises and diet tips, with each chapter exploring different aspects of hormonal balance for optimal well-being.

This is your comprehensive resource that holds tools and information grounded in scientific research and real-life experience. As a blend of guide, journal, and recipe book, you will find plenty of pertinent and helpful content, all while indulging in gentle reflective practices and discovering delicious foods to reset your gut and nervous system. In other words, the guide itself provides actionable steps, the journal invites you to reflect and track progress, and the recipe book invites you to try new nourishing meals to support your mind and body.

One more thing: I know time is precious. I also know that past experiences may have left you cautious. You might think, "I've tried detox plans before, and they didn't work." Know that the following chapters have been designed to address those concerns, one by one. It is a work crafted to fit into your life, so please, take your time and be kind to yourself along the way. You don't need to overhaul everything overnight. Small, consistent changes lead to lasting results.

I can assure you that by implementing the strategies outlined here, you can expect tangible benefits. Improved energy levels, balanced hormones, and reduced stress are within reach.

Thank you for joining me on this journey. Also, I hope you know that your body will be most grateful for this huge dose of self-care. Together, let's explore the path to better health and well-being. Embrace the opportunity to transform your life, one step at a time. Your journey begins now, and I am honored to be part a part of it.

ONE
UNDERSTANDING CORTISOL AND ITS IMPACT

ON A SEEMINGLY ORDINARY MORNING, you might find yourself rushing through breakfast, coffee in hand, already feeling the pull of the day ahead. By afternoon, you're battling fatigue and frustration, wondering why your energy feels so depleted. It's a familiar scenario, one that's all too common for many caught up in the whirlwind of modern life. At the core of this reality lies cortisol, a hormone that plays a pivotal role in how your body handles stress and maintains balance. As we navigate this chapter, we will uncover the deep and fascinating ties between cortisol and our health, unlocking secrets that lead to equilibrium and renewed energy.

The Cortisol Connection

Cortisol is a remarkable hormone produced by the adrenal glands, small but mighty organs perched atop your kidneys. It serves as one of the body's essential regulators, orchestrating a number of functions that keep you balanced. When you face stress, your body releases cortisol as part of its fight-or-flight response, preparing you to tackle challenges head-on. This hormone also maintains your blood pressure, ensuring that your circulatory system operates smoothly. Beyond these roles, cortisol supports your immune system, playing a central role in your body's defense against illness and inflammation. However, when cortisol levels become imbalanced, the ripple effects can impact every facet of your health.

This hormone doesn't work in isolation; it dances alongside other hormones like estrogen and progesterone, especially significant in women's health. These interactions are particularly evident during the menstrual cycle. Fluctuations in cortisol can amplify mood swings and cognitive challenges, leaving you feeling out of sync. The balance between these hormones is delicate, and disruptions can manifest as irritability or difficulty concentrating. Grasping this concept is important, as it sheds light on how stress can extend its reach, spiraling into wider health issues and influencing your mental and emotional state.

When cortisol levels stray too far from the norm, the consequences can be far-reaching. High cortisol can lead to adrenal fatigue, where your body's stress response becomes blunted, leaving you exhausted and vulnerable. Chronic elevation of cortisol is linked to an array of chronic diseases, from cardiovascular issues to metabolic disorders. Conversely, insufficient cortisol can compromise your body's ability to respond to stress, making everyday challenges feel insurmountable. Maintaining balance is therefore vital for safeguarding your health and vitality.

The significance of regulating cortisol levels cannot be overstated. Emerging studies shed light on how influential balanced cortisol is for our resilience to stress and overall health enhancement. For example, a systematic review has illuminated the benefits of mindfulness and relaxation practices in moderating cortisol levels, opening up effective pathways for managing stress. Further, investigations into the hormonal shifts experienced during menopause have pinpointed the impact of biological changes on cortisol balance, showing the necessity of personalized strategies in achieving hormonal equilibrium. These findings affirm the role of mindful cortisol management as a foundation for comprehensive wellness.

Understanding cortisol's multifaceted role will allow you to appreciate its significance in your life. So much more than a stress hormone, it plays a key role in your body, influencing everything from immune function to mood regulation.

How Stress and Cortisol Shape Our Daily Life

FOR MOST OF US, every morning, stress begins to weave its web. As we prepare for the day ahead, the demands of work, household responsibilities, social obligations and family duties form a complex (and familiar) rhythm that our bodies respond to with precision. As stressors mount, cortisol levels rise, setting off a chain reaction. This hormone, released by our adrenal glands, prepares our body to face perceived threats. It's a survival mechanism, but in today's world, the threats are more likely to be deadlines and family obligations than predators. The cycle of stress and cortisol becomes a familiar pattern, impacting our bodies in ways we might not immediately recognize.

In the average lives of women aged 35 to 55, stress will manifest in numerous ways. Careers often peak during these earlier years, bringing both opportunities and pressures. Balancing professional ambitions with family life can feel like walking a tightrope. The physiological response to stress is automatic: cortisol floods your system, increasing your heart rate, sharpening your senses, and preparing your muscles to react. While this response is beneficial in short bursts, chronic stress keeps cortisol levels elevated over long periods. This constant flood leaves you wired yet tired, affecting your focus, productivity, and relationships.

Imagine (or, perhaps you don't even need to imagine) managing a work presentation while your child's school calls with an issue.

Your focus splinters, and irritability creeps in. Elevated cortisol clouds your cognitive functions, making it hard to concentrate. You might snap at a colleague or, later, misinterpret a partner's words. Stress reactions stimulate cortisol production, influencing how you connect with others. As you've surely noticed, hormonal turbulence can lead to mood swings, where minor inconveniences feel insurmountable. The cycle perpetuates, as stress breeds more stress, pulling you deeper into its grasp.

Breaking this cycle requires intentional shifts in daily mind and body habits, which we will now begin to explore alongside each topic. When tackling the "mind" aspect of cortisol detox, a good place to start is with short mindfulness practices like a few minutes of deep breathing or meditation. These also provide much-needed moments of calm amidst life's chaos. Establishing boundaries is another powerful tool, albeit not always an easy one to implement at once. However, allocating specific times for work and personal life - including "me" time - creates a buffer that will allow you to recharge. This separation prevents stress from bleeding into every corner of our existence, which tends to happen without us even realizing how much it is impacting every facet of our life. By making space for yourself, you will grant your body the chance to reset, reducing cortisol and restoring balance.

Journaling: 30 Days of Mindful Moments

Understanding the stress-cortisol cycle equips us with the knowledge to reclaim control. Set aside five minutes each day, morning or evening, to sit quietly. Focus on your breath, allowing your thoughts to drift by without judgment, and jot down your thoughts. In order to develop this reflective habit, I invite you to use the following template in your journal to track your mindful moments over the course of thirty days. This simple practice will help center your mind and set a peaceful tone for the day.

Date:

Mindful Thoughts:

Emotions and feelings that arise:

Practice Observations:

The Midlife Cortisol Surge

AS WE NAVIGATE THROUGH MIDLIFE, our body undergoes a series of transformative hormonal shifts, marking a significant phase in our life. During this period, women experience the onset of perimenopause, gradually transitioning into menopause. This transition brings about changes in hormonal production, most notably a fluctuation in estrogen and progesterone levels. Midlife thus becomes a time when cortisol levels often surge, adding another layer of complexity to the physical and emotional changes you're already managing. Increased cortisol can make us more susceptible to stress, amplifying feelings of tension and anxiety. This heightened stress response leads to a cascade of effects, including weight gain, particularly around the abdomen, as your metabolism adjusts to the new hormonal environment. The change in hormones during this stage often feels daunting, but understanding these will equip you with the knowledge to navigate them more effectively.

It's clear that the implications of heightened cortisol during midlife extend beyond stress and weight. Prolonged exposure to elevated levels can pose risks to cardiovascular health. High cortisol levels have been linked to increased blood pressure and a greater likelihood of developing heart disease. The stress hormone's impact on our cardiovascular system underscores the importance of addressing hormonal imbalances during this critical life stage. As we contend with these physiological changes, it becomes most crucial to seek balance, not only for physical health but for our overall quality of life.

Achieving hormonal harmony during midlife requires a multifaceted approach, one that addresses both nutrition and lifestyle - hence the nature of this handbook. A diet rich in nutrients that support hormonal balance will certainly help mitigate the effects of cortisol. Foods high in omega-3 fatty acids, such as salmon and flaxseeds, have anti-inflammatory properties that can help regulate hormone levels. Similarly, consuming whole grains and legumes provides your body with essential fiber, aiding in the stabilization of blood sugar levels, which in turn supports cortisol management. We'll dive into this further as we continue.

It has also been found that integrative health approaches further complement nutritional strategies. Practices such as yoga and meditation not only reduce stress but also promote a sense of calm and well-being. These practices encourage mindfulness, allowing us to reconnect with our body and mind to help us navigate hormonal shifts. Additionally, regular exercise tailored to personal preferences and physical capabilities enhances our body's ability to manage stress and regulate cortisol. So, really, it's about finding what resonates with you, and creating a routine that feels sustainable and supportive of your unique needs.

Understanding these dynamics empowers us to make informed choices that align with our health goals, ensuring that we thrive during this potentially beautiful transformative phase. As you learn about these strategies, you will cultivate an environment where hormonal harmony can flourish, offering a path toward balance amidst the changes of midlife.

Cortisol's Role in Weight Gain and Energy Depletion

Amidst the everyday rhythm of life, cortisol silently directs the complex ballet of energy management and fat storage within your body. When finely balanced, it ensures a seamless metabolic performance. Yet, when stress levels chronically rise, cortisol's role shifts, leading to metabolic imbalances that often surface as weight gain. The connection between cortisol and insulin resistance becomes evident as your body starts to falter in its glucose processing capabilities. This inefficiency prompts an increase in fat storage, especially around the midsection, initiating a difficult-to-break cycle. The altered distribution of fat exacerbates the problem, as the body opts to conserve energy rather than expend it, creating a persistent battle with weight management.

Traditional diets often overlook the critical role of cortisol in weight gain. They tend to focus on calorie counting or rigorous exercise, which tend to inadvertently heighten stress and, ironically, cortisol levels. The link between cortisol and insulin resistance becomes apparent when the body begins to struggle with processing glucose efficiently. This resistance prompts your body to store more fat, creating a cycle that's challenging to break. Altered fat distribution then compounds the issue, as the body prioritizes storing energy rather than burning it, leading to a persistent struggle with weight management.

Hence, adopting a cortisol-conscious eating strategy is essential. Such plans highlight foods that stabilize blood sugar, including whole grains and lean proteins, and embrace healthy fats like avocados and nuts. These dietary choices help regulate cortisol levels, leaving us with a metabolic environment in balance.

Furthermore, with sustained high levels of cortisol, the pathways of energy production are also compromised. Chronic elevation of this hormone can leave us feeling perpetually tired, devoid of energy regardless of how much rest you attempt to get. This is in part due to disrupted sleep patterns. Cortisol levels are supposed to decrease at night to facilitate restful sleep, but when stress keeps them elevated, it leads to a night of restless sleep instead of rejuvenating rest. This deterioration in sleep quality further drains your energy, perpetuating a vicious cycle of fatigue. Beyond affecting sleep, cortisol also hampers the way our cells generate and utilize energy, making each day feel like an uphill battle.

To effectively address the interconnected challenges of cortisol regulation, weight management, and sustained energy levels, you might want to explore adaptogenic herbs such as ashwagandha (Withania somnifera) and rhodiola (Rhodiola rosea). Adaptogens are natural substances that help the body maintain homeostasis under stress by modulating the hypothalamic-pituitary-adrenal axis and supporting adrenal function.

Ashwagandha has been shown to reduce cortisol levels significantly, improve sleep quality, and enhance resilience to stress. For instance, randomized controlled trials suggested that daily supplementation with ashwagandha can lower serum cortisol by up to 30%, which may contribute to reduced stress-induced weight gain and better metabolic health.

Rhodiola, on the other hand, is known for its energizing properties. It is known to improve physical performance, reduce fatigue, and promote mental clarity by influencing key stress-response pathways, including the regulation of stress-induced oxidative damage and inflammation. A dose of 200–600 mg per day has been shown to be effective in clinical settings.

Incorporating these herbs as part of a balanced diet—via teas, tinctures, or standardized supplements—can provide a scientifically-supported, natural approach to mitigating the effects of chronic stress. Also, remember to consult a healthcare professional before starting any new supplement regimen, especially if you have underlying health conditions or are on medication.

Recipes: Easy Adaptogenic Herb Concoctions

Adaptogenic herbs have long been celebrated for their ability to help the body adapt to stress, balance hormones, and enhance overall well-being. In this section, you will find simple and effective recipes to incorporate these powerful plants into your daily routine. Each recipe is designed to support cortisol detox, promote hormonal balance, aid weight loss, and improve mind-body harmony.

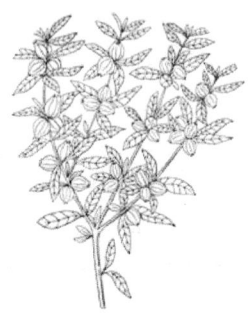

Golden Adaptogen Latte

Ingredients:

- 1 cup unsweetened almond milk (or milk of choice)
- 1/2 tsp turmeric powder
- 1/2 tsp ashwagandha powder
- 1/4 tsp cinnamon powder
- 1 tsp honey or maple syrup (optional)
- Pinch of black pepper
- 1/4 tsp vanilla extract (optional)

Instructions:

1. Heat the almond milk in a small saucepan over low-medium heat.
2. Add turmeric, ashwagandha, cinnamon, and black pepper. Whisk well to combine.
3. Remove from heat and stir in honey and vanilla extract, if using.
4. Pour into a mug and enjoy warm, preferably in the evening for a calming effect.

Morning Adaptogen Smoothie

Ingredients:

- 1 banana (fresh or frozen)
- 1/2 cup frozen berries (blueberries or strawberries work well)
- 1 cup unsweetened coconut water or plant-based milk
- 1/2 tsp maca powder
- 1/2 tsp reishi mushroom powder
- 1 tbsp almond butter or sunflower seed butter
- 1/4 tsp ground ginger (optional for added zest)

Instructions:

1. Add all ingredients to a blender.
2. Blend on high speed until smooth and creamy.
3. Pour into a glass and drink as a nutrient-packed breakfast or pre-workout snack.

Adaptogenic Herbal Tea Infusion

Ingredients:

- 2 cups boiling water
- 1 tsp dried holy basil (tulsi)
- 1/2 tsp dried rhodiola root
- 1/2 tsp dried licorice root
- 1/2 tsp dried lemon balm (optional for flavor)
- Honey or lemon to taste (optional)

Instructions:

1. Combine the herbs in a teapot or heatproof jar.
2. Pour boiling water over the herbs and cover.
3. Steep for 10-15 minutes, then strain.
4. Sweeten with honey or add a splash of lemon, if desired. Drink warm or chilled.

THE COMPLETE CORTISOL DETOX HANDBOOK

Adaptogen Bliss Balls

Ingredients:

- 1 cup pitted Medjool dates
- 1/2 cup raw almonds or walnuts
- 1/4 cup unsweetened shredded coconut
- 1 tbsp cacao powder
- 1 tsp ashwagandha powder
- 1 tsp maca powder
- 1 tbsp chia seeds
- 1-2 tbsp almond butter

Instructions:

1. Add all ingredients to a food processor and blend until the mixture comes together into a sticky dough.
2. Roll into small balls (about 1 inch in diameter).
3. Optional: Roll the balls in shredded coconut or cacao powder for extra flavor.
4. Store in an airtight container in the refrigerator for up to 1 week.

Adaptogen-Infused Lemonade

Ingredients:

- 1 cup filtered water
- Juice of 1 fresh lemon
- 1/2 tsp powdered ginseng or rhodiola
- 1 tsp raw honey or agave syrup
- A pinch of Himalayan pink salt
- Ice cubes (optional)

Instructions:

1. In a glass, mix the powdered adaptogen with a small amount of warm water to dissolve.
2. Add lemon juice, honey, and salt.
3. Pour in the remaining water and stir well.
4. Add ice cubes if desired, and enjoy this refreshing drink during midday for an energy boost.
5. Each recipe in this section not only delivers health benefits but also makes your adaptogenic routine enjoyable and delicious. Adjust ingredient quantities to suit your personal taste and health goals.

Emotional Well-being: Cortisol's Silent Influence

In quiet moments when you find yourself grappling with the ebb and flow of emotions, cortisol is often a silent player directing your mood. It subtly influences your emotional landscape, contributing to feelings of anxiety or depression, and at times creating a rollercoaster of emotions that seem to arise without warning. It's as if your emotional thermostat has been tampered with, causing sudden spikes or dips that leave you feeling out of control. Emotional dysregulation becomes a frequent companion, where balancing between calm and chaos feels like a constant struggle. This disruption is not just psychological; cortisol affects neurotransmitter balance, altering the levels of chemicals in the brain that regulate mood and emotions. It's a delicate dance, and when cortisol leads, the rhythm can become unsettling, making it challenging to find your emotional footing.

Building emotional resilience in the face of cortisol's influence will require a toolkit of strategies designed to fortify your mental armor. Cognitive-behavioral strategies offer a powerful means of reframing negative thought patterns, allowing us to shift our perspective and respond to stress with greater ease. By identifying and challenging the thoughts that feed anxiety, we create space for more balanced emotions. Developing emotional intelligence is another key component. This involves understanding our emotional triggers and learning to navigate them with empathy and self-awareness. This consists of recognizing the signals our body sends and responding with compassion rather than judgment. Such skills are invaluable in managing the emotional upheavals that cortisol can provoke.

Furthermore, support systems play a pivotal role in maintaining emotional health. The bonds we form with family, friends, and community members act as a buffer against the stresses of life. Engaging in community activities not only provides a sense of belonging but also offers opportunities to share experiences and gain perspective. Building a support network is like weaving a safety net, one that can catch us during moments of emotional freefall.

By nurturing these connections and embracing strategies for emotional resilience, we create a foundation for enduring well-being. This journey is deeply personal, yet universally shared. It is about creating an environment where cortisol's influence is acknowledged and managed, ensuring that emotional health remains a priority.

Emotional Well-Being Checklist

Emotional health plays a vital role in managing cortisol levels and achieving overall well-being. Use this list to regularly assess and nurture your emotional state as part of your cortisol detox journey.

Daily Practices for Emotional Balance

- **Practice Gratitude**: Write down three things you're grateful for today.
- **Engage in Positive Self-Talk**: Replace negative thoughts with empowering affirmations.
- **Set Daily Intentions**: Start your day by setting an intention to cultivate calm and positivity.
- **Deep Breathing or Meditation**: Spend 5–10 minutes focusing on your breath or meditating to center yourself.
- **Connect with Nature**: Spend at least 10–15 minutes outdoors, soaking in natural light and fresh air.

Stress Management

- **Identify Stress Triggers**: Take note of moments when you feel stressed and the situations that cause them.
- **Establish Healthy Boundaries**: Say no to commitments that overwhelm you and prioritize self-care.
- **Move Your Body**: Engage in gentle exercises like yoga, walking, or stretching to release tension.

- **Schedule Relaxation Time**: Dedicate time each day to unwind, whether through reading, a hobby, or a calming bath.

Emotional Check-Ins

- **Rate Your Emotions**: On a scale of 1–10, how do you feel emotionally today?
- **Acknowledge Your Feelings**: Accept and name your emotions without judgment.
- **Practice Emotional Release**: Journal, cry, or vent to release built-up emotions.
- **Focus on the Present Moment**: Use mindfulness to anchor yourself in the here and now.

Healthy Relationships

- **Communicate Effectively**: Express your thoughts and needs clearly and kindly.
- **Nurture Supportive Connections**: Spend time with friends or family who uplift and inspire you.
- **Avoid Toxic Interactions**: Limit contact with people or situations that drain your energy.
- **Give and Receive Love**: Share acts of kindness, hugs, or words of affirmation with loved ones.

Sleep and Emotional Regulation

- **Create a Relaxing Evening Routine**: Limit screen time and engage in calming activities before bed.

- **Journal Before Sleep**: Reflect on your day and release worries to prevent overthinking at night.
- **Prioritize Rest**: Aim for 7–9 hours of quality sleep each night to restore emotional resilience.

Celebrating Wins

- **Acknowledge Progress**: Celebrate small achievements, even if they seem minor.
- **Reward Yourself**: Treat yourself to something special when you reach personal milestones.
- **Practice Self-Compassion**: Be gentle with yourself on tough days—progress isn't always linear.

Self-Reflection Prompts

- *What brought me joy today?*
- *What challenges did I face, and how did I respond?*
- *What is one thing I can do tomorrow to feel more emotionally balanced?*

Recognizing High Cortisol Levels: Signs and Symptoms

Within the fluctuations of daily life, cortisol can quietly stir disruptions, signaling its presence through an array of symptoms that often blend into the backdrop of busy routines. Persistent weight gain, particularly when it seems resistant to diet and exercise, is a common indicator that something is amiss. As we've discussed, this weight often settles around the abdomen, a telltale sign of cortisol's influence. As the days unfold, you might notice an undercurrent of anxiety or a quick temper, even in situations where you typically feel composed. This shift can cause irritability to creep into interactions, straining relationships and leaving you wondering why patience feels like a distant memory. Sleep disturbances further complicate the picture. Nights that should offer respite instead bring restless tossing and turning, as cortisol levels refuse to decrease, robbing you of much-needed rest.

To better understand these symptoms, some diagnostic tools can offer clarity. Salivary cortisol testing provides a non-invasive method to assess cortisol levels at various points throughout the day, capturing the natural peaks and troughs of this hormone. Blood tests, though more invasive, deliver precise measurements that can confirm whether cortisol levels have strayed from their normal range. Interpreting these results can be complex, as cortisol's rhythm fluctuates regularly. A healthcare professional will be able to guide you through understanding what these numbers mean and how they relate to your symptoms.

Self-awareness is another powerful (and often underestimated) ally in recognizing and addressing cortisol imbalances. Keeping a symptom diary can truly help pinpoint patterns and triggers. By noting when you experience certain symptoms, alongside daily stressors or lifestyle choices, you will begin to see connections that might otherwise go unnoticed. Reflecting on these entries can reveal insights into how your lifestyle impacts your hormonal health, shedding light on areas ripe for adjustment. This practice will enhance your understanding while equipping you with valuable information to track your health.

It goes without saying that when symptoms persist despite lifestyle changes, you should aim to seek professional guidance. Consulting a healthcare practitioner experienced in hormonal health is a highly helpful and effective method of tackling hormonal imbalances head-on. Endocrinologists, who specialize in hormone-related conditions, are particularly well-equipped to interpret complex hormonal interactions. Your GP should be able to guide you through this process; however, you may want to prepare for these consultations by gathering relevant information, including your symptom diary and any test results you've obtained. Medical specialists who have a comprehensive view of your health are more able to provide tailored recommendations that align with your unique needs.

Cortisol Fluctuations: Symptom Diary

This symptom diary template is designed to help you track daily fluctuations in your cortisol levels and their effects on your hormonal balance, weight, mental clarity, and overall well-being. By observing patterns, you can gain valuable insights into your body's responses and fine-tune your holistic detox plan.

Daily Symptom Log

Date: _____

Time of Entry: _____

Morning (Upon Waking)

- **Energy Level (1-10):** _____
- **Mood (e.g., calm, anxious, irritable):** _____
- **Physical Symptoms (e.g., fatigue, stiffness, bloating):** _____
- **Hunger Level (1-10):** _____
- **Sleep Quality (1-10):** _____
- **Notes on Dreams/Rest:** _____

Midday (Around Noon)

- **Energy Level (1-10):** _____
- **Mood:** _____
- **Physical Symptoms:**
  _____
- **Hunger Level (1-10):** _____
- **Stressors/Triggers (if any):**
  _____
- **Cognitive Function (e.g., clarity, focus):**
  _____

Afternoon (Around 4 PM)

- **Energy Level (1-10):** _____
- **Mood:** _____
- **Physical Symptoms:** _____
- **Hunger Level (1-10):** _____
- **Stressors/Triggers:** _____
- **Cravings (if any):** _____

Evening (Before Bed)

- **Energy Level (1-10):** _____
- **Mood:** _____
- **Physical Symptoms:** _____
- **Hunger Level (1-10):** _____
- **Sleep Preparation (e.g., rituals, relaxation methods):** _____

- **Overall Stress Level (1-10):**
  _____

Daily Reflection

What went well today?

Challenges faced and possible triggers:

Adjustments for tomorrow:

Overall Cortisol Impact Rating (1-10): _____

Weekly Review Section
(To be completed at the end of each week)

Key Patterns Observed:

Triggers Noted:

Most Effective Stress Management Strategies:

Areas for Improvement:

TWO

THE SCIENCE OF DETOXIFICATION

DETOXIFICATION IS AN AGE-OLD NATURAL PROCESS, our body's method of expelling toxins and maintaining equilibrium. Contrary to popular belief, it does not require extreme diets or drastic measures, but instead relies on supporting the body's innate ability to cleanse itself. This essential function helps us handle environmental pollutants, dietary byproducts, and the effects of daily stress, ensuring optimal health and equilibrium.

At the core of detoxification lie the liver and kidneys, your body's silent warriors. The liver, often referred to as the body's chemical laboratory, converts harmful toxins into less harmful substances, making them easier for your body to eliminate. It diligently produces bile to assist digestion and processes nutrients to energize your body. Meanwhile, your kidneys meticulously filter the blood, expelling waste and excess substances through urine. Together, these organs form a formidable team, ensuring toxins are efficiently processed and expelled before they can cause systemic damage. Their effectiveness is crucial for maintaining health and averting the accumulation of toxins, which can lead to various health complications.

As you may have guessed, detoxification goes far beyond eliminating toxins. For one thing, it significantly impacts cortisol management. By diminishing inflammation, a natural consequence of stress and toxin exposure, detoxification supports the regulation of cortisol levels. This regulation is essential since chronic inflammation can upset hormonal balance, triggering heightened stress responses. Thus, effective detoxification facilitates the reduction of inflammation, setting the stage for improved hormonal stability. When your body functions optimally, with inflammation under control, cortisol levels stabilize, which creates a sense of physical and emotional equilibrium.

The ripple effects of detoxification extend past hormonal balance. As toxins are efficiently expelled and inflammation is reduced, you'll notice an uptick in energy levels. This rejuvenation boosts physical vitality while permeating your mental clarity. With a reduced toxic load, brain fog lifts, enhancing your ability to think clearly and concentrate on daily activities. This clarity can revolutionize your life experience, making even mundane moments more vivid and engaging. When your body functions with fewer toxins, everything from digestion to mood can see significant improvement.

I suggest you take a moment to jot down your current habits. Perhaps there are some modifications you could make to encourage detoxification. Pause to reflect on how these adjustments might integrate into your daily routine and how they could enhance your overall well-being. This is a wonderful opportunity for you to step in and take the lead, mainly by removing obstacles in order to allow your body to function at its best. There are plenty of ways in which you can support your body's built-in cleansing system, designed to handle the challenges of a modern lifestyle filled with environmental pollutants and daily stresses.

Detoxification should be perceived not as a fleeting endeavor but as a way of life—a continual practice that bolsters long-term health. This lifestyle includes integrating detox-supportive habits into your everyday routine. Simple adjustments, such as drinking

THE SCIENCE OF DETOXIFICATION

ample water, consuming a diet abundant in whole foods, and reducing processed foods, can make a substantial difference. You'll want to approach these habits in a sustainable way, ensuring that each change harmonizes with your lifestyle and supports your body's natural processes without overwhelming it. Remember that overwhelm tends to create stress, therefore increases cortisol production, which would be quite counterproductive. Try to embrace detox as a lifestyle by committing to small, consistent practices that enhance lasting health and resilience.

Detoxification Habits Checklist

Reflecting on your habits is an essential part of maintaining hormonal balance and supporting your body's natural detoxification processes. Use this checklist to identify areas for growth and to celebrate the habits you're already implementing.

1. Prioritize Hydration

- Drink at least 8-10 glasses of water daily to support kidney function and flush out toxins.
- Include hydrating foods like cucumbers, watermelon, and celery in your diet.
- Consider adding a pinch of mineral-rich sea salt or a splash of lemon juice to your water for added electrolytes.

2. Embrace Anti-Inflammatory Foods

- Incorporate more leafy greens, cruciferous vegetables, and colorful fruits rich in antioxidants.
- Use spices like turmeric, ginger, and cinnamon to reduce inflammation and enhance detox pathways.
- Minimize processed foods, sugar, and trans fats to support optimal liver function.

3. Support Gut Health

- Include probiotic-rich foods such as yogurt, kefir, sauerkraut, or miso.
- Eat fiber-rich foods like oats, lentils, chia seeds, and artichokes to promote regular elimination.

- Limit artificial sweeteners and highly processed foods that disrupt gut flora.

4. Encourage Daily Movement

- Aim for 30 minutes of moderate exercise daily, such as walking, yoga, or cycling, to stimulate lymphatic flow.
- Integrate strength training or high-intensity interval training (HIIT) to enhance metabolism and hormonal health.
- Practice restorative exercises like stretching or tai chi to support stress reduction.

5. Focus on Restorative Sleep

- Create a calming bedtime routine with activities like reading, meditation, or gentle stretches.
- Avoid screens and caffeine at least two hours before bed.
- Keep your bedroom cool, dark, and quiet to improve sleep quality.

6. Practice Stress-Reduction Techniques

- Dedicate time to mindfulness or meditation practices to lower cortisol levels.
- Spend time in nature to reduce stress and reset your nervous system.
- Engage in journaling or creative activities that bring you joy and peace.
- Seek out opportunities to laugh and enjoy pleasant moments.

7. Detox Your Environment

- Replace conventional cleaning products and cosmetics with non-toxic alternatives.
- Reduce exposure to plastics by using glass, stainless steel, or silicone containers.
- Incorporate indoor plants like peace lilies or snake plants to improve air quality.

8. Nourish with Targeted Supplements (Consult a Professional)

- Consider supplements like milk thistle, dandelion root, or NAC (N-acetylcysteine) to support liver detox.
- Include adaptogens like ashwagandha or holy basil to help manage stress and support hormonal health.
- Ensure adequate intake of vitamins D, B-complex, and magnesium for overall well-being.

Reflect and Act

As you review this checklist, choose two to three habits to focus on this week. Reflect on how these changes make you feel and consider journaling your progress. Remember, small, consistent steps lead to transformative results over time. You've got this!

THE SCIENCE OF DETOXIFICATION

Your Body's Natural Detox Pathways

Our bodies are somewhat similar to a bustling city, where each organ plays a specific role in keeping things running smoothly. The liver, kidneys, digestive tract, skin, and respiratory system are the vital organs that work tirelessly to detoxify your body. The liver, often referred to as the body's powerhouse, takes center stage by breaking down and neutralizing toxins, thus preventing them from wreaking havoc. It processes everything from alcohol to medications, ensuring that harmful substances are transformed into less harmful ones. Meanwhile, the kidneys act as meticulous gatekeepers, filtering blood to remove waste products and excess substances, which are then expelled through urine. The digestive tract plays its part by excreting waste, while the skin and lungs expel toxins through sweat and breath. These organs work together in a harmonious system, each contributing its part to the detoxification process, keeping the body healthy and balanced.

All of these detox pathways work together. The liver and gut collaborate closely, with the liver processing toxins and the gut ensuring their safe passage out of the body. The lymphatic system, often overlooked, plays an important role in transporting waste products away from tissues, acting as a clean-up crew that ensures your body stays clean and efficient. This system helps to remove cellular debris and other waste, supporting the immune system and maintaining fluid balance. So, when one pathway struggles or becomes overwhelmed, others compensate, highlighting the resilience and adaptability of our body's detoxification network. The seamless operations between these systems is vital, as it ensures a smooth flow of detoxification, preventing the accumulation of harmful substances that can disrupt your health.

Supporting these systems is key to enhancing your body's natural detox capabilities. As you know, hydration should always be at the forefront of your mind as it is fundamental to healthy bodily functions. Water serves as the medium through which toxins are flushed out. Drinking plenty of water aids the kidneys in filtering and excreting waste, while also keeping the skin hydrated and promoting healthy digestion. Aim to drink at least eight glasses a day, and perhaps think about incorporating herbal teas like chamomile or peppermint, which not only hydrate but also offer soothing properties for digestion and stress relief.

Again, a diet rich in whole foods, including fruits, vegetables, lean proteins, and whole grains, provides essential nutrients that support liver function and overall detoxification. These foods supply vitamins and minerals that act as cofactors in detoxification processes, ensuring that your body has the tools it needs to perform optimally. By making these dietary choices, you provide your body with the building blocks necessary for effective detoxification.

You may also want to think about progressively eliminating certain habits from your lifestyle, which will allow the detoxification process to take place. Alcohol and smoking are an added burden on the liver and lungs, requiring them to work harder to eliminate toxins. Reducing or eliminating these can relieve stress on your detox pathways, allowing them to function more efficiently.

Regular exercise, on the other hand, boosts detoxification by promoting circulation and lymphatic drainage. Physical activity encourages sweating, which helps expel toxins through the skin, and enhances the efficiency of the respiratory and cardiovascular systems. By including regular movement into your routine, you will support your body's natural detox processes and contribute to overall health.

In summary, your lifestyle choices have a significant impact on these detox pathways. These choices are within your control. In time, they become habits that have a significant lasting effect on your body's ability to detoxify and maintain balance.

Preparing Your Body for Detox

EMBARKING on a detox requires more than just a decision. This huge act of self-care inevitably involves preparing both mind and body for the process ahead.

A good place to begin is by setting realistic expectations. Understand that detoxification is not an overnight miracle, but a gradual change that relies on sustainable positive habits. You may wish to start with mental preparation techniques, which can be as simple as mindfulness or journaling. Take a few moments each day to visualize your health goals and the steps you'll take to achieve them. This mental clarity will ground your efforts and keep you motivated. Emotionally, it's essential to embrace the journey with an open mind, allowing yourself to adapt and learn as you proceed.

As you prepare mentally, consider the dietary changes that will ease your transition into detox. A simple way to start is by eliminating processed foods, which are often loaded with preservatives, artificial additives, unhealthy fats, and high levels of sugar and sodium. These ingredients can strain your body's detoxification systems, disrupt gut health, and contribute to inflammation, metabolic imbalances, and long-term health issues such as obesity, heart disease, and diabetes. Opt for whole foods that are closer to their natural state, like fresh fruits, vegetables, and whole grains. These provide essential nutrients and fiber that support your body's natural detox processes.

You might also want to gradually reduce caffeine and sugar, which can spike cortisol levels and disrupt your body's equilibrium. Again, let me emphasize that this process must be slow and gradual to ensure that minimal stress ensues. Instead of going cold turkey, ease these out to minimize withdrawal symptoms and allow your body to adjust smoothly. This measured and subtle reduction will allow your body to begin detoxification while also stabilizing your energy levels. This reduces the peaks and crashes associated with these substances. Moreover, it supports emotional and mental balance throughout the process, creating a holistically proactive approach.

Rest must also be seriously considered as it directly influences your body's ability to regulate stress hormones and support detoxification. Without proper rest, cortisol levels can remain elevated, undermining your detox efforts and overall health. Therefore, establishing optimal sleep habits is essential. Aim for at least 7 hours of uninterrupted, high-quality sleep each night to allow your body sufficient time to recover and regenerate. Create a calming bedtime routine that avoids screens, stimulants, and stressors to signal your body that it's time to wind down. Remember, deep, restorative sleep is when many critical processes occur, including hormone regulation, tissue repair, and the activation of the glymphatic system, which clears waste products from the brain.

Additionally, preparing for detox involves a few practical steps to ensure you're fully equipped. Stock up on whole foods, which will be the foundation of your detox diet. Fill your pantry with essentials like legumes, nuts, seeds, and a variety of colorful produce. These foods will support your body's nutritional needs and keep you satisfied throughout the process. Also, take time to identify potential detox triggers in your environment—these could be anything from stressors at work to unhealthy snacks in your kitchen. By recognizing these triggers, you can create strategies to avoid or manage them, further smoothing your detox path. This preparation phase is about creating a supportive environment that aligns with your health goals, setting you up for a successful detox experience.

Potential Detox Triggers

EMBARKING on a cortisol detox plan and striving for hormonal balance requires a keen awareness of the environmental factors that may undermine your progress. Your surroundings—physical, emotional, and digital—can significantly influence your stress levels and overall well-being.

Go through each of the following categories systematically, noting any triggers present in your environment. For each identified trigger, create an actionable plan to reduce or eliminate its impact. Remember, the goal is not perfection but progress. Small, consistent changes will create a ripple effect that enhances your cortisol detox and promotes lasting hormonal balance.

Environmental Toxins

- Household Products: Check for cleaning supplies, air fresheners, and detergents containing harsh chemicals. Opt for natural or eco-friendly alternatives.
- Plastics: Avoid storing food and drinks in plastic containers, especially if they are not BPA-free. Replace them with glass, stainless steel, or silicone options.
- Personal Care Items: Examine skincare, makeup, and hair products for endocrine-disrupting chemicals like parabens, phthalates, and synthetic fragrances.
- Air Quality: Assess for sources of indoor air pollution such as mold, dust, or chemical fumes. Consider investing in air purifiers and incorporating houseplants to improve air quality.

Dietary Stressors

- Processed Foods: Identify packaged snacks and meals high in refined sugars, trans fats, and artificial additives.

- Caffeine Overload: Monitor your coffee, tea, and energy drink intake to avoid overstimulating your adrenal glands.
- Pesticides: Choose organic produce when possible, or thoroughly wash conventional fruits and vegetables.
- Food Sensitivities: Track potential intolerances or allergens, such as gluten, dairy, or soy, that may trigger inflammation or hormonal imbalance.

Digital Stressors

- Screen Time: Reflect on how much time you spend on screens, especially before bed. Excessive exposure to blue light can disrupt your circadian rhythm.
- Social Media: Evaluate your relationship with social media. Are certain platforms or interactions leaving you anxious, stressed, or drained?
- Notifications: Disable non-essential alerts that interrupt your focus and contribute to chronic stress.

Emotional Triggers

- Toxic Relationships: Identify connections that consistently leave you feeling depleted or overwhelmed.
- Unresolved Stressors: Pinpoint situations or memories causing lingering tension. Consider journaling, therapy, or meditation to process these feelings.
- Overcommitment: Assess your calendar for over-scheduling. Prioritize rest and activities that nourish your well-being.

Physical Environment

- Clutter: Review your living and working spaces for clutter. A tidy, organized environment promotes calm and clarity.
- Lighting: Check for harsh fluorescent lighting. Incorporate warm-toned light bulbs or natural sunlight to create a soothing ambiance.
- Noise Pollution: Identify sources of disruptive noise and use soundproofing techniques or white noise machines as needed.

Myths and Misconceptions

Detoxification is often shrouded in myths that can mislead and even harm those of us looking to improve our health. One of the most common misconceptions is that detox is a quick fix, promising rapid weight loss or instant health improvements. This belief can lead to a cycle of unrealistic expectations and disappointment. As we have previously discussed, detoxification should always be viewed as a sustained practice, not a magic bullet.

The idea that detox requires extreme fasting is another prevalent myth. While some people swear by fasting as a method to cleanse the body, it's not the only path to detoxification, and it can sometimes do more harm than good. Scientific studies show that, in some instances, fasting can slow metabolism. In these cases, the body switches to a conservation mode to preserve energy, which can counteract weight loss efforts in the long run. Don't get me wrong: Different types of fasting can offer a range of benefits, including improved mental clarity, enhanced metabolism, better digestion, and support for cellular repair and overall well-being. Moreover, there are highly effective intermittent fasting techniques that are gentle on the body while delivering positive results. It must, however, follow regular patterns that allow the body to gently adapt, without provoking extreme feelings of deprivation. In fact, research on safe detox practices highlights the importance of balanced approaches. Studies indicate that gradual dietary adjustments are more effective and sustainable than drastic measures. The emphasis should be on supporting our body's natural detox processes rather than overloading it with extreme changes.

The harm of adhering to misleading detox methods can be significant. Choosing to follow extreme diets or fasting regimens without professional guidance can lead to nutrient deficiencies, depriving the body of essential vitamins and minerals needed for optimal health. This deprivation can weaken the immune system, making you more susceptible to illness. Furthermore, the psychological stress of following unrealistic detox plans can create a negative relationship with food and body image, leading to cycles of guilt and frustration – not to mention an increase in cortisol levels.

Therefore, informed decision-making is key to navigating the world of detoxification safely and effectively. Consulting with various healthcare professionals can provide personalized guidance that aligns with your health goals and medical history. They can help you tailor a detox plan that supports your body's needs without compromising your well-being. Personalized approaches are important to consider, because what works for one person may not be suitable for another. By taking into account your lifestyle, dietary preferences, and health conditions, you can develop a plan that is both effective and enjoyable, two factors that also influence cortisol levels.

Evidence-Based Detox Techniques for Women

ALTHOUGH DETOXIFICATION IS OFTEN MISUNDERSTOOD, when rooted in scientifically-supported methods, it can be a powerful tool

THE SCIENCE OF DETOXIFICATION

for enhancing well-being. One approach gaining traction is intermittent fasting, which involves cycling between periods of eating and fasting. This method allows the body time to reset and repair, promoting cellular repair processes and enhancing metabolic health. Studies suggest that intermittent fasting can help reduce inflammation and improve insulin sensitivity, making it a valuable practice for managing cortisol levels. To determine which type of intermittent fasting is best for you, you'll want to consider your lifestyle, daily schedule, and health goals, as well as factors such as your energy needs, any medical conditions, and how your body responds to periods of fasting. Again, consulting with a healthcare professional can also help ensure safety and effectiveness. Overall, intermittent fasting will give your digestive system a break, which will allow your body to focus on detoxification and energy conservation.

Nutrition itself plays a pivotal role in detoxification. Vegetables like broccoli, kale, and Brussels sprouts are particularly beneficial for liver support. These veggies contain compounds that enhance liver enzyme production, helping to neutralize and eliminate toxins. Antioxidant-rich foods, such as berries, nuts, and dark leafy greens, combat oxidative stress, reducing cellular damage and supporting the body's natural detox processes. Add these foods into your meals to create a strong defense against the daily onslaught of environmental toxins, all while supporting your body's ability to maintain hormonal balance.

Furthermore, holistic practices complement nutritional strategies and enhance detoxification outcomes. Mind-body therapies, including yoga and tai chi, promote relaxation and reduce stress, both of which are crucial for effective detoxification. These practices encourage mindfulness, allowing you to tune into your body's needs and respond with care. Mindfulness meditation is also a powerful tool that helps to lower cortisol levels by developing a sense of calm and presence. Regular practice can improve emotional regulation and boost resilience, making it easier to navigate stress without overwhelming your system.

Incorporating detox techniques into your daily routine can be simple and effective. Start your day with a morning lemon water ritual—squeeze fresh lemon juice into a glass of warm water to kickstart digestion and support liver function. This simple habit not only hydrates but also flushes out toxins accumulated overnight. In the evening, embrace relaxation practices such as a warm bath infused with Epsom salts or essential oils. This time will allow your body to unwind, contributing to better sleep and recovery.

Implementing probiotics into your diet is another strategy worth considering. These beneficial bacteria support gut health, which is integral to the detoxification process. A healthy gut flora aids digestion and enhances the elimination of waste, reducing the toxic burden on your liver. Probiotics can be found in fermented foods like yogurt, kefir, and sauerkraut, or in supplement form. Regular consumption can improve digestive health and bolster your body's natural defenses.

These evidence-based techniques offer a solid baseline for effective detoxification, supporting a harmonious balance between body and mind. By integrating these practices into your lifestyle, you will begin to create a foundation for enduring health and vitality, empowering yourself to face life's challenges with enhanced emotional resilience and mental clarity.

Tailoring Detox

DETOXIFICATION ISN'T A ONE-SIZE-FITS-ALL ENDEAVOR. Your body, lifestyle, and health conditions are unique, and your detox plan should reflect that individuality. Personalizing your detox plan is key to its success. If you have specific health conditions, such as thyroid disorders or diabetes, your approach needs to be carefully tailored. Consulting with a healthcare provider will help you understand how detoxification may interact with your current health status and medications. This step ensures that your detox plan supports rather than disrupts your health. Additionally, consider your daily routine and responsibilities. Whether you're balancing a hectic work schedule, family obligations, or personal commitments, your detox plan should fit seamlessly into your life. Make gradual changes that align with your existing lifestyle, allowing for a smoother transition and greater adherence to the plan.

Personal preferences also play a role in how effectively you stick to a detox plan. Choose methods that resonate with you. If you find joy in plant-based diets, incorporate them into your detox plan. If you're drawn to specific physical activities like swimming or cycling, make them a regular part of your regime. Engaging in activities you enjoy increases the likelihood of maintaining the detox process and keeps cortisol levels in check. When the methods you choose align with your preferences, you're more likely to view them as a lifestyle rather than a temporary change or, even worse, as an additional stressor. This mindset shift is key to long-term success and makes the detox experience more enjoyable and rewarding.

Tracking your progress is another essential aspect of personalizing and optimizing your detox plan. Journaling can be a powerful tool for self-reflection, helping you identify patterns and triggers that influence your health. By writing down your daily experiences, dietary changes, and emotional states, you will gain valuable insights into what works and what doesn't. Health tracking apps can also be beneficial, offering a convenient way to monitor your food intake, physical activity, and even sleep patterns. These tools provide a visual representation of your progress, making it easier to identify areas for improvement and celebrate your achievements. The data you collect can guide adjustments to your plan, ensuring it remains effective and aligned with your goals.

As for ongoing evaluation and adaptation, make sure to set periodic reassessment dates to review your progress and make necessary adjustments. This practice ensures that your plan evolves with your changing needs and circumstances. Seeking feedback from health professionals can provide additional guidance, helping you refine your approach and address any challenges you encounter. Regularly reviewing and tweaking your plan will keep it dynamic and responsive, preventing stagnation and promoting continuous improvement. This proactive approach is empowering as it makes us take control of our health, leading with informed decisions that support our own well-being.

As you leap onto the path of detoxification, remember that flexibility and personalization are your allies. By tailoring your plan to fit your unique needs and preferences, you will create a sustainable framework for long-term health. This approach transforms detox from a daunting task into an empowering journey, one that aligns with your life. With a personalized plan, you will be well-equipped to discover the plethora of detoxification benefits.

THREE
NUTRITION FOR HORMONAL HARMONY

Last Sunday morning, under a blazing summer sun, I wandered into the chaos of my local farmer's market—packed with people, bursting with color, and absolutely drowning in the smell of fresh bread and sweet mangoes. I paused at a stall brimming with fresh produce, marveling at the vivid reds of ripe tomatoes and the deep greens of kale. In that grounding moment, I was reminded that it's here, amidst nature's bounty, that we have the power to transform our health. Such a simple thing – yet, so often overlooked. In these basic natural foods lies the key to harmonizing our hormones and reducing the relentless grip of cortisol. Therefore, if we learn to embrace the power of nutrition, we can nourish our bodies and restore balance within, even in a world that often feels overwhelming.

Anti-Inflammatory Foods: Allies in Cortisol Reduction

Inflammation is a term that often conjures images of swelling or pain, yet it plays a more insidious role in your body's stress response. When chronic inflammation takes hold, it puts undue stress on your adrenal glands, which are responsible for producing cortisol. This creates a vicious cycle where inflammation begets stress, and stress begets more inflammation. Fortunately, anti-inflammatory foods can break this cycle. Omega-3 fatty acids, found abundantly in fatty fish like salmon and in plant sources like flaxseeds, are potent inflammation fighters. These healthy fats support heart health while also soothing inflammation, helping to keep cortisol levels in check.

Berries and leafy greens are nutritional powerhouses, teeming with antioxidants that combat oxidative stress and inflammation. Blueberries, for instance, contain anthocyanins, compounds that not only give them their vibrant hue but also confer protective effects against cellular damage. Spinach and kale are rich in vitamins A, C, and E, as well as phytonutrients that bolster your body's defenses. By adding these foods to your diet, you will arm yourself against the daily onslaught of stressors that elevate cortisol. The science is clear: reducing inflammation can significantly impact cortisol production, making these foods indispensable in your quest for hormonal harmony.

Among the most celebrated anti-inflammatory foods are turmeric and ginger. Turmeric's active compound, curcumin, has been studied extensively for its anti-inflammatory properties. It can inhibit inflammatory pathways at the molecular level, offering relief from chronic inflammation and its associated ailments. Similarly, ginger, often used in traditional medicine, contains gingerol, a compound that reduces inflammation and promotes digestive health. Adding these spices to your meals not only enhances flavor but also provides a robust defense against inflammation. They're versatile enough to be used in teas, soups, and stir-fries, making them easy to incorporate into your daily routine.

Adding these anti-inflammatory foods to your diet won't require a complete overhaul of your eating habits. Simple changes can make a big difference. You can start your day with overnight oats or a smoothie packed with chia seeds, berries, and spinach; the

NUTRITION FOR HORMONAL HARMONY

seeds add a satisfying texture and are rich in omega-3s. Dress your salads with 1 tablespoon of extra virgin olive oil, a healthy fat that complements fresh vegetables while providing additional anti-inflammatory benefits. These small, delicious adjustments can seamlessly integrate into your lifestyle, enhancing both your meals and your health.

Anti-Inflammatory Food Checklist

When aiming to detox for stress and inflammation reduction, the right foods can work wonders. Use this checklist of anti-inflammatory foods that you may choose to include in your weekly shopping. Note your favorites and experiment with new recipes to keep meals exciting and nutritious.

Fruits

- **Berries** (blueberries, strawberries, raspberries): Rich in antioxidants and vitamin C to combat stress-induced inflammation.
- **Oranges and Grapefruits**: High in vitamin C, which lowers cortisol levels.
- **Cherries**: Contain melatonin and anti-inflammatory compounds to promote restful sleep and recovery.
- **Bananas**: Provide potassium to regulate blood pressure during stress.

Vegetables

- **Leafy Greens** (spinach, kale, Swiss chard): Packed with magnesium, which helps relax the body and regulate cortisol.
- **Broccoli**: Contains sulforaphane, a compound known to reduce inflammation and support detoxification.
- **Sweet Potatoes**: High in beta-carotene and fiber, which stabilize blood sugar and reduce stress.
- **Avocado**: Loaded with healthy fats and potassium to combat stress and lower cortisol.

Healthy Fats

- **Olive Oil**: Rich in omega-3s, which are essential for reducing inflammation.
- **Nuts and Seeds** (walnuts, almonds, flaxseeds, chia seeds): Provide healthy fats, protein, and magnesium.
- **Fatty Fish** (salmon, mackerel, sardines): High in omega-3 fatty acids to reduce stress and inflammation.

Protein Sources

- **Eggs**: A versatile source of high-quality protein and choline, supporting brain health and hormonal balance.
- **Turkey and Chicken**: Lean proteins that help stabilize blood sugar levels and reduce cortisol spikes.
- **Lentils and Chickpeas**: Plant-based protein rich in B vitamins to support energy and stress regulation.

Spices and Herbs

- **Turmeric**: Contains curcumin, a powerful anti-inflammatory compound.
- **Ginger**: Supports digestion and reduces inflammation.
- **Cinnamon**: Balances blood sugar levels to minimize cortisol fluctuations.
- **Chamomile and Peppermint**: Herbal teas that promote relaxation and calm.

Whole Grains and Complex Carbs

- **Quinoa**: A complete protein and complex carbohydrate that supports steady energy release.

- **Oats**: High in soluble fiber and stress-reducing compounds.
- **Brown Rice**: Provides magnesium and helps maintain a stable mood.

Beverages

- **Green Tea**: Contains L-theanine, which promotes relaxation without drowsiness.
- **Matcha**: A powdered green tea with calming properties and antioxidants.
- **Bone Broth**: Rich in collagen and minerals to support gut health and reduce stress.

Snacks and Extras

- **Dark Chocolate** (70% cacao or higher): Boosts serotonin and reduces cortisol levels.
- **Greek Yogurt**: Packed with probiotics to support gut health and balance hormones.
- **Fermented Foods** (sauerkraut, kimchi, kefir): Promote a healthy gut microbiome, which is crucial for stress resilience.

Quick Tips for Incorporating These Foods:

- Create salads using leafy greens, berries, and avocado.
- Cook with anti-inflammatory spices like turmeric and ginger.
- Snack on nuts, seeds, or a piece of dark chocolate for a quick stress-busting boost.
- Prepare warm, comforting soups with bone broth, lentils, and a medley of vegetables.

NUTRITION FOR HORMONAL HARMONY

- Swap sugary beverages for herbal teas or green tea to maintain a calm and focused state of mind.
- Add fatty fish like salmon or sardines to meals for a dose of omega-3s that help combat inflammation.
- Blend smoothies with ingredients like spinach, flaxseeds, berries, and almond milk for a nutrient-packed start to your day.
- Use olive oil or avocado oil instead of vegetable oils when cooking to reduce inflammatory fats.
- Add fermented foods like sauerkraut, kimchi, or yogurt to your meals
- Choose whole grains like quinoa, buckwheat, or brown rice over refined grains to stabilize blood sugar.

Meal Planning for Hormonal Balance

PREPARING meals that satisfy hunger and support hormonal balance begins with understanding macronutrients—protein, fats, and carbohydrates—and how they work together to maintain balance. Each macronutrient plays an important role: protein helps in repairing tissues and maintaining muscle mass, healthy fats support hormone production, and carbohydrates provide the energy needed to power through your day. Fiber is equally important, as it regulates hormones by stabilizing blood sugar levels and aiding digestion. By structuring your meals to include a balance of these nutrients, you will create a foundation for hormonal harmony.

If your goal is to minimize stress and ensure a nutritious diet, effective meal planning is your ally. Batch cooking saves time and energy by allowing you to prepare larger quantities of food in advance, so you can enjoy a home-cooked meal even on your busiest days. A good approach is to dedicate a weekend afternoon to cooking a few staple dishes that you can mix and match throughout the week. Plus, meal prepping means you'll dodge the dreaded "What's for dinner?" debate and the last-minute stress trip to the grocery store, where you go in for one thing and somehow leave with a cart full of snacks. When planning your meals, take some time to source seasonal ingredients. These add variety and ensure that you're getting the freshest, most nutrient-rich produce available, often at a lower cost, which is a bonus for your wallet.

Creating a meal plan that fits your lifestyle doesn't have to be complicated. For breakfast, think about options that combine protein and healthy fats, like an avocado toast with a poached egg or a smoothie bowl topped with nuts and seeds. These meals are quick to prepare and keep you full and energized for hours. For lunch, focus on nutrient-dense choices like a quinoa salad with grilled chicken, mixed greens, and a sprinkle of seeds. Add a simple olive oil and lemon dressing for a flavorful and nutritious boost.

Planning ahead ensures that each meal is both satisfying and supportive of your health goals.

Of course, meal planning can come with its own set of challenges, particularly when time and budget are factors. Quick meal preparation techniques, such as using a slow cooker or an instant pot, can be lifesavers. These devices allow you to prepare meals with minimal effort, freeing up your time for other activities. When it comes to budget concerns, cost-effective shopping tips are essential. Start by making a list before heading to the grocery store and stick to it to avoid impulse purchases. Buying in bulk, especially when it comes to pantry essentials like grains and legumes, can lead to significant savings over time. Additionally, consider swapping out some expensive ingredients for more affordable alternatives without compromising on nutrition.

Adaptogens in Diet: Nature's Stress Relievers

ADAPTOGENS ARE like whispers of secret ancient wisdom, natural herbs that hold the power to support your body's resilience to stress. They are unique in that they help regulate your body's stress response, particularly through their impact on cortisol levels. Ashwagandha, one of the most well-known adaptogens, has been shown to reduce cortisol levels significantly. It's a staple in Ayurvedic medicine, offering a gentle, yet effective way to calm the mind and body. Meanwhile, Rhodiola, often found in the arctic regions, is known for enhancing resilience to stress, boosting energy, and improving mood.

Using adaptogens can be as simple as enjoying a warm cup of tea or adding a spoonful of powder to your smoothie. Maca powder, derived from a root native to the high Andes of Peru, is a fantastic addition to morning smoothies. It not only adds a rich, nutty flavor but also supports energy levels and hormonal balance. Holy basil, another revered adaptogen, can be brewed into a soothing tea.

Often referred to as tulsi, this herb is celebrated for its ability to reduce stress and promote mental clarity. Sipping on holy basil tea can become a comforting ritual, providing a moment of calm in a busy day.

The efficacy of adaptogens is supported by a growing body of research. Various clinical trials have demonstrated their ability to lower stress markers and improve psychological well-being. Studies show that Withania somnifera, the scientific name for ashwagandha, significantly decreases serum cortisol levels and reduces perceived stress in adults. These findings show the potential of adaptogens to offer a natural alternative to conventional stress management methods. By normalizing cortisol levels, adaptogens help restore balance to the hypothalamic–pituitary–adrenal axis, which is often disrupted by chronic stress.

While adaptogens are generally safe, it's important to approach them with care and awareness. Possible interactions with medications can occur, particularly with herbs like Rhodiola and ashwagandha. For instance, some may cause gastrointestinal discomfort or interact with antidepressants and anticoagulants. Therefore, consulting with a healthcare provider before adding adaptogens to your diet will ensure that you choose the best options for your individual needs. Medical professionals in tune with holistic healthcare methods can provide guidance on appropriate dosages and help you understand any potential side effects. By taking these precautions, you can safely enjoy the benefits of nature's stress relievers, safely integrating them as a supportive element in your wellness plan.

Gut Health and Cortisol

YOUR GUT CONTAINS trillions of microorganisms, known as the gut microbiota, which play a key role in keeping your body functioning properly. These microorganisms help regulate hormones, including cortisol.

The gut-brain axis is the communication highway between your digestive system and your brain, and it is this connection that influences your stress levels and overall well-being. When stress hits, your body releases cortisol, which impacts digestive health, leading to a cycle of discomfort and imbalance. Chronic stress can disrupt the delicate balance of gut bacteria, contributing to issues like bloating and irregular bowel movements.

Let's explore this further. A healthy gut microbiota helps regulate hormone levels, including cortisol, which creates a more resilient system to handle stress. The gut and brain communicate through the gut-brain axis, a complex network involving the nervous system, immune signals, and microbial metabolites like short-chain fatty acids (SCFAs). Certain beneficial bacteria, such as Lactobacillus and Bifidobacterium species, can modulate the hypothalamic-pituitary-adrenal (HPA) axis, reducing excessive cortisol release during stressful situations. Additionally, a balanced gut flora supports the production of serotonin, a neurotransmitter linked to mood regulation, further enhancing the body's ability to cope with stress effectively.

I'm sure you've heard about probiotics and prebiotics. These stand at the forefront of maintaining gut wellness, and consequently, achieving a balanced cortisol level. Probiotics are live beneficial bacteria that support a healthy gut flora, improving digestion, nutrient absorption, and the gut-brain communication essential for regulating stress responses. Common sources of probiotics include fermented foods such as yogurt, kefir, sauerkraut, kimchi, miso, and kombucha. Adding a variety of these foods in your diet is sure to enhance the diversity and resilience of your gut microbiome.

Prebiotics, on the other hand, are non-digestible fibers that serve as nourishment for these beneficial bacteria, helping them thrive and multiply. Foods rich in prebiotics include garlic, onions, leeks, asparagus, bananas, and whole grains. Combining prebiotics and probiotics—known as synbiotics—can maximize their benefits, supporting a strong and balanced gut microbiome.

Now, improving gut health will necessitate thoughtful dietary and lifestyle changes. Including fermented foods, such as sauerkraut, kimchi, and miso, in your meals will introduce beneficial bacteria to your gut. These foods are delicious and support digestion by helping to maintain balance within the microbiome. Reducing processed food intake, as we have previously discussed, is another important and unavoidable step. Processed foods contain preservatives and artificial ingredients that can disrupt gut health and exacerbate stress-related digestive issues. So, opting for whole, unprocessed foods will enhance your gut function and health. Additionally, staying hydrated and engaging in regular physical activity will further boost the health of your digestive system.

As you prepare for a gut detox or begin to implement changes, you should lookout for signs of digestive imbalance to address gut health issues promptly. Symptoms like persistent bloating, irregular bowel movements, and unexplained fatigue can indicate that your gut may need some extra attention. Paying attention to these signals and seeking professional advice when necessary can prevent minor issues from becoming major concerns. Again, work with your healthcare provider. Having this support can help you identify underlying causes and develop a plan to restore balance, all while having your personal health and wellness goals in mind. Often, small changes that we hadn't considered ourselves – such as specific dietary adjustments or supplements to support gut health – can go a long way in managing hormones and stress effectively.

Recipes for Relaxation

STEPPING into the kitchen has often been my refuge from the chaos of the day, a space where I can slow down and engage in a form of culinary meditation. I have no doubt that the act of cooking allows us to immerse ourselves in the present, focusing on tactile sensations such as the slicing vegetables or the rhythmic stirring of a simmering pot. I particularly love that this mindful process can transform meal preparation into a therapeutic activity, offering a respite from stress. Creating a calming kitchen environment further enhances this experience. Using soft lighting and playing gentle music to set a soothing tone can have a huge impact on the mindfulness component of this once-mundane task. Let your kitchen become a safe and peaceful space where you can unwind and nurture yourself through the simple act of concocting healthy meals.

As far as preserving inner calm goes, adding certain ingredients to your recipes can further amplify the stress-relieving benefits of cooking. Imagine savoring a dessert infused with chamomile, its floral notes providing a gentle lull to your senses. Chamomile, known for its relaxing properties, can be mixed into a light pudding or delicate cake. Pairing this with a lavender and lemon balm tea creates a tranquil finish to your meal, as the aromatic herbs work together to reduce cortisol levels and promote relaxation. These recipes delight the palate and soothe the mind, transforming your whole dining experience into a holistic practice of self-care.

The dining experience itself also plays a role in nurturing calm and relaxation. You can choose to set your table with calming colors, such as soft blues or gentle greens, which can create a peaceful atmosphere. Adding elements like scented candles or fresh flowers can further enhance the ambiance, turning a simple meal into a mindful ritual. These thoughtful touches invite you to pause and appreciate the moment, allowing you to fully engage with your food and the present. When you create a space that invites relaxation, every meal becomes an opportunity to reconnect with yourself and find peace amidst the noise of daily life.

Meals are more than just a source of nourishment—they are an opportunity for connection and emotional well-being. In today's fast-paced world, taking the time to sit down and share a meal with others can be a powerful way to slow down and recharge. Sharing meals with loved ones not only deepens a sense of connection but also has measurable benefits for both mental and physical health, including nervous system regulation and stress management. Eating slowly and mindfully during shared meals activates the parasympathetic nervous system, or "rest-and-digest" mode, which helps lower cortisol levels, reduce stress, and improve digestion. The calming rhythm of chewing, savoring food, and engaging in conversation encourages a state of relaxation, supporting both physical and emotional well-being.

Additionally, the act of gathering around a table allows for meaningful connections and a sense of safety, which further regulates the nervous system and promotes emotional resilience. Socializing while eating stimulates the release of feel-good hormones like oxytocin and serotonin, helping to counteract the negative effects of stress. This practice has been linked to improved heart health, stronger immune function, and better mental clarity.

Whether it's a family dinner or a casual meal with friends, shared meals offer an opportunity to slow down, connect, and recharge. These moments are invaluable. They nourish the body with food but also nourish the soul with human connection, helping to manage stress and regulate emotions.

Avoiding Dietary Pitfalls: Foods That Spike Cortisol

IN THE HUSTLE of daily life, the choices made at the grocery store or the coffee shop quietly influence how you feel throughout the day. Cortisol is sensitive to what we consume. Foods and drinks that might seem harmless can elevate cortisol levels, exacerbating stress and its effects on the body. Caffeine, found in coffee and energy drinks, is a well-known stimulant. It certainly has many benefits such as heightening alertness and temporarily boosting

NUTRITION FOR HORMONAL HARMONY

energy, but it also triggers the release of cortisol. For many, a morning cup of coffee is a ritual, yet its impact on stress hormones can linger, especially if consumed in large quantities. Similarly, high-sugar snacks, often tempting in moments of fatigue or stress, cause blood sugar levels to spike and crash. This rollercoaster effect prompts the body to release more cortisol to stabilize blood sugar, setting off a cycle that can leave you feeling more stressed and drained than before.

Your dietary habits have a huge impact on how your body manages stress, particularly through their influence on blood sugar levels. Skipping meals, whether due to a busy schedule or an effort to cut calories, can cause blood glucose levels to drop, depriving the brain of the steady energy it needs to function optimally. In response, the body will release cortisol to help stabilize energy levels. This can lead to feelings of irritability, fatigue, and difficulty concentrating. Over time, chronically low or erratic blood sugar levels can contribute to heightened stress sensitivity and hormonal imbalances. Similarly, consuming processed foods high in refined sugars and unhealthy fats causes rapid spikes and crashes in blood glucose. These fluctuations strain our body's ability to maintain balance. In fact, they downright elevate cortisol levels, impairing our capacity to handle stress effectively.

Fortunately, there are healthier dietary options that can help manage stress and boost energy levels without sacrificing enjoyment. Gradually reducing your daily coffee intake is a good start, and swapping your morning coffee for herbal teas like chamomile or peppermint can offer a calming and caffeine-free alternative. Yes, parting ways with your beloved morning coffee might feel like an emotional breakup at first, but these teas can help lower cortisol levels, promote relaxation, and gently energize your body—without the jittery rollercoaster or the mid-morning crash that has you reaching for a second (or third) cup.

For a more indulgent yet health-conscious option, we have the trending adaptogenic hot chocolates, which combine cacao with herbs like ashwagandha, reishi, or maca. This adaptogenic concoction is designed to support stress management, enhance focus, and sustain energy without the jittery effects of caffeine. Cacao itself is rich in magnesium, which aids in relaxation and muscle function, while also containing natural compounds that improve mood and boost mental clarity.

Furthermore, when cravings strike, reaching for whole fruits instead of sugary desserts can provide natural sweetness along with fiber, vitamins, and minerals to stabilize blood sugar and maintain energy. Pairing fruits with healthy fats, like almond butter or yogurt, further help regulate energy levels throughout the day. Moderation remains essential, as even natural sugars can affect blood sugar if consumed in excess.

Mindful eating is another popular strategy that can help curb cortisol spikes. Practicing portion control, for instance, allows you to enjoy your favorite foods without overindulgence. By being aware of how much you eat, you can prevent the discomfort and stress that often follow overeating. Mindfulness extends beyond portions; it also involves savoring each bite. Taking the time to truly taste and enjoy your food can enhance satisfaction and reduce the urge to consume more than necessary. This encourages a deeper connection with your meals and a greater awareness of how food affects your body and mind.

Avoiding dietary pitfalls is not about strict deprivation but about making informed choices that support your body's natural rhythms. By identifying foods that spike cortisol and embracing healthier alternatives, you will support your body in managing stress more effectively. These changes create a balanced relationship with food, one that nourishes both body and soul. As you continue to explore the role of nutrition in hormonal harmony, remember that every small choice contributes to your overall health.

FOUR
EXERCISE AND MOVEMENT FOR STRESS REDUCTION

Exercise. The word alone might make you want to fake an injury and dramatically collapse onto the couch. But hear me out—movement doesn't have to mean sweating buckets in a gym or attempting a yoga pose that looks like a human pretzel gone wrong. Something as simple as a walk around the neighborhood can do wonders for your well-being. It helps reduce stress, clears your mind, and—bonus—gives you an excuse to eavesdrop on your neighbors' questionable landscaping choices. I know that the moment my feet hit the pavement, my worries start to fade with every step. It's not just movement; it's a scientifically proven way to trick your brain into chilling out. Exercise is so much more than burning calories or building muscle; it's one of the best tools for managing stress, balancing hormones, and, let's be honest, justifying that post-walk snack.

Finding the right exercise routine is essential to harnessing these benefits. Different activities affect cortisol levels in unique ways, and personalizing your exercise choices is key. What works for one person might not suit another. Enjoyment plays a crucial role here; when you find joy in movement, it becomes a source of pleasure rather than a chore. This enjoyment helps maintain consistency, which is vital to achieving long-term goals and sustainable stress management. Matching the intensity of your workouts with your personal stress levels is also very important. For some, high-intensity workouts provide a necessary release, while others might find calm through lower-intensity, steady-state activities. Ultimately, the right fit is one that aligns with your lifestyle and emotional needs, one that allows you to exercise in a way that feels both rewarding and sustainable.

Exercise and cortisol have an intricate relationship. Short bursts of high-intensity exercise, such as sprinting or interval training, can initially spike cortisol levels due to the immediate stress placed on the body. However, over time, these activities can lead to improved stress resilience and lower baseline cortisol levels. On the other hand, aerobic exercises like walking, cycling, or swimming offer a more moderate approach. These are renowned for their calming effects, reducing stress through physiological and psychological mechanisms. According to Harvard Health Publishing, aerobic exercise lowers stress hormones like cortisol and increases endorphins, those feel-good chemicals that boost mood and provide a natural sense of relaxation.

So, where to begin? Choosing the right exercise often requires a bit of exploration. Experimenting with different classes or sports can help identify what resonates with you. If you're unsure where to start, there are flexible options like fitness apps that provide opportunities to explore new activities from the comfort of your home. These tools offer a variety of workouts, allowing you to try everything from dance to strength training without a long-term commitment. As you sample different exercises, pay attention to how each makes you feel, both physically and mentally. This awareness can guide you toward activities that not only fit your schedule but also enhance your mood and energy levels.

Adding movement and exercise to your daily life doesn't have to be a grand affair. Once more, let's remember that simple changes

EXERCISE AND MOVEMENT FOR STRESS REDUCTION

can make a significant difference. For example, scheduling walking meetings can be a good way to combine work and exercise. Desk exercises during breaks are also easy yet highly beneficial routine adjustments. Small actions, like taking the stairs instead of the elevator or parking a little farther from your destination, can add up to meaningful movement throughout the day. These adjustments will make it easier to stay active without disrupting your responsibilities.

Exercise Preference Quiz

This quick quiz will help you identify your exercise preferences to better manage stress and support your emotional, physical, and mental well-being. Your results should guide you toward activities that align with your lifestyle and wellness goals.

1. How active are you currently?

- A. I'm mostly sedentary, with minimal physical activity.
- B. I engage in light activity, like occasional walks or yoga.
- C. I'm moderately active and enjoy regular workouts.
- D. I'm very active, exercising intensely several times a week.

2. What intensity level do you prefer in exercise?

- A. Gentle and calming (e.g., stretching, yoga, tai chi).
- B. Moderate and steady (e.g., walking, cycling, dance).
- C. Energizing but manageable (e.g., strength training, Pilates).
- D. High-energy and intense (e.g., running, HIIT, spin classes).

3. What type of activities do you enjoy?

- A. Mind-body practices (e.g., yoga, meditation, breathing exercises).
- B. Outdoor activities (e.g., hiking, gardening, walking).
- C. Group or social activities (e.g., dance classes, team sports).
- D. Competitive or goal-oriented workouts (e.g., races, personal records).

4. What is your main goal for incorporating exercise?

- A. To relieve stress and feel calmer.
- B. To improve energy and overall health.
- C. To build strength or tone muscles.
- D. To challenge myself and see measurable progress.

5. How much time can you realistically dedicate to exercise?

- A. 15–20 minutes a few times a week.
- B. 30–45 minutes on most days.
- C. 1 hour or more for focused sessions.
- D. I can adjust my schedule to fit intense or lengthy workouts.

6. What type of environment do you prefer for exercise?

- A. At home with minimal equipment.
- B. Outdoors in nature or open spaces.
- C. In a gym or fitness class with others.
- D. Anywhere, as long as it's dynamic and exciting.

7. How do you typically feel after exercising?

- A. Relaxed and recharged.
- B. Energized but not overworked.
- C. Satisfied and accomplished.
- D. Exhilarated and ready for more.

8. Do you like to track progress or set fitness goals?

- A. Not really—I focus more on how I feel in the moment.
- B. I keep it simple, like counting steps or time spent moving.
- C. Yes, I enjoy tracking improvements like strength or endurance.
- D. Absolutely! I thrive on metrics and setting ambitious goals.

Results and Recommendations

COUNT how many times you selected A, B, C, or D to find your primary exercise type:

Mostly A's: You thrive on gentle, restorative movements. Activities like yoga, tai chi, or light stretching can help reduce stress and promote mental clarity.

Mostly B's: You enjoy balanced, moderate activities. Walking, cycling, or dancing are ideal for improving health while keeping things fun and sustainable.

Mostly C's: You prefer energizing and structured exercises. Try strength training, Pilates, or swimming to build strength and maintain a steady routine.

Mostly D's: You're motivated by intensity and challenges. Activities like running, HIIT, or competitive sports can help you channel energy and meet goals.

Mindful Movement: Yoga and Pilates for Stress Relief

If you've ever practiced yoga, you might be familiar with the ritual of gently unfurling your mat in a quiet corner of your living room. A certain feeling of peace washes over you as the soft light filtering through the curtains eases your mind and body into a gentle practice. Yoga and Pilates, with their roots in mindful movement, are disciplines that focus on breathwork and alignment, creating a harmonious flow that soothes the nervous system. In yoga, the breath acts as a guide, connecting the pieces of our being through each movement to cultivate balance and calm. Pilates, with its emphasis on core strength and flexibility, extends this mindfulness to every controlled movement, inviting us to connect deeply with our body's innate wisdom. These practices create a powerful antidote to the stress that can accumulate in daily life, providing a pathway to holistic restoration.

Mindful movement practices have been proven to be effective for somatic recovery and stress regulation, particularly by modulating cortisol production. Both yoga and Pilates activate the parasympathetic nervous system, counterbalancing the heightened sympathetic activity associated with chronic stress and excessive cortisol secretion. This shift creates a state of relaxation, reducing the physiological wear-and-tear caused by prolonged activation of the hypothalamic-pituitary-adrenal axis.

The benefits of including yoga and Pilates into your routine extend beyond the mat. Engaging in these mindful movement practices can lead to a significant reduction in muscle tension, offering relief from the physical manifestations of stress. As you stretch and strengthen, you release built-up tension, allowing your muscles to relax and your posture to improve. This physical release is mirrored in the mind, where mental clarity and focus are enhanced. Through the meditative aspects of yoga and Pilates, it is possible to cultivate a sense of inner stillness, quieting the mental chatter that

EXERCISE AND MOVEMENT FOR STRESS REDUCTION

often accompanies stress. This clarity tends to spill over into daily life, making it easier to handle challenges with grace and ease.

Moreover, regular yoga practice has been shown to attenuate cortisol output by engaging mechanisms such as vagal stimulation through deep, diaphragmatic breathing and meditative focus. These techniques suppress the stress response while improving heart rate variability, an important biomarker for resilience to stress. Lower cortisol levels directly correlate with reduced inflammation, improved glucose metabolism, and better cognitive function, making yoga a highly effective intervention for both mental and physical health.

Pilates complements these effects by enhancing proprioception, muscular balance, and core strength, which reduces physical tension that often exacerbates stress-related symptoms. The precise, controlled movements inherent in Pilates improve neuromuscular efficiency, further aiding in somatic recovery. Both practices promote the release of endorphins and serotonin, bolstering mood and mental clarity while mitigating the cognitive fog often associated with dysregulated cortisol levels.

For those new to these practices, starting with beginner-friendly routines can ease the transition. In yoga, a basic sun salutation sequence offers a gentle introduction. This flowing series of postures moves through forward folds, lunges, and upward stretches, guided by the rhythm of your breath. It awakens the body and calms the mind, setting a peaceful tone for the day. In Pilates, introductory mat exercises focus on building foundational strength and flexibility. Simple movements, such as pelvic tilts and leg lifts, engage the core and enhance body awareness. These routines require minimal equipment, making them accessible for practice at home, and they can be adapted to suit individual fitness levels and needs.

Combining mindfulness with movement practices significantly enhances their stress-relief and overall health benefits, as supported by research in neuroscience and physiology. When mindfulness is applied during exercise, it activates the parasympathetic nervous system, tapping into a state of calm and reducing cortisol levels. Powerful calming techniques like diaphragmatic breathing and alternate nostril breathing (nadi shodhana) can also be used in yoga, Pilates, or even strength training to enhance focus and relaxation.

Moreover, mindful movement encourages heightened interoception—the awareness of internal bodily sensations—leading to improved body alignment, injury prevention, and a deeper connection between mind and body. Studies also show that combining mindfulness with physical activity increases the release of endorphins and modulates the default mode network in the brain, increasing present-moment awareness and reducing rumination. This beneficial approach supports stress management while boosting mood, enhancing performance, and promoting long-term adherence to exercise routines.

You will also find that visualization practices during poses invite you to imagine tension melting away or energy flowing freely, enhancing the meditative quality of the exercise. During poses or movements, employing visualization techniques—such as imagining tension dissipating like smoke or energy coursing through the body like a flowing river—activates neural pathways associated with relaxation and focus. It also reinforces motor learning and proprioception by helping the brain rehearse and refine movements, even in static poses. This dual engagement of mental imagery and physical action deepens the meditative aspect of exercise. Regular practice can reduce stress while training your brain to remain anchored in the present, creating a ripple effect of improved focus and emotional regulation in daily life.

Cardio with Care: Balancing Intensity and Relaxation

Let me start by confessing something: I have never been a runner.

In fact, for most of my life, the closest I came to running was a panicked dash to grab the last avocado at the farmer's market. Yet somehow, recently, I've found myself jogging—yes, jogging—through a peaceful park near my home. No music, no podcasts, just the rhythmic thud of my feet on the path, occasionally interrupted by the chattering of an overly confident kookaburra. At first, I was certain I'd hate it, half-expecting my legs to rebel and my lungs to stage a dramatic protest. But oddly enough, these quiet moments have started to grow on me, becoming not just tolerable but oddly therapeutic—a surprising ally in the ongoing battle against anxiety and overthinking. Who knew the path to inner peace might involve so much sweat?

Cardiovascular exercise actually plays a dual role in stress management, acting as both a stress reliever and, if overdone or poorly managed, a potential stressor. High-intensity cardiovascular workouts are particularly effective for enhancing mental and physical resilience because they trigger the release of endorphins and other neurochemicals like dopamine and serotonin, which elevate mood and reduce stress. This type of exercise also improves heart rate variability, a marker of vagus nerve health and a key indicator of a well-regulated stress response.

Exercising in a social context—such as team sports or group fitness classes—amplifies these benefits by combining physical activity with the positive effects of social connection. Engaging with others during exercise increases feelings of camaraderie and trust, which are vital for regulating the nervous system. Social interactions stimulate the vagus nerve, which plays a central role in the parasympathetic "rest-and-digest" state, countering the effects of chronic stress.

Moreover, when fun and laughter are part of workouts, the stress response is further modulated by lowering cortisol levels and increasing feelings of joy and engagement. These elements make exercise more sustainable and ensure that the physical benefits are matched by mental and emotional gains, creating a holistic approach to stress management that supports both short-term relief and long-term wellness.

Now, for most, moderate-intensity cardio is where the sweet spot lies. This level is both effective and sustainable, as it offers the benefits of endorphin release and improved mood without overwhelming your body.

Moderate-intensity workouts, typically performed at 50–70% of your maximum heart rate, help release endorphins without causing excessive strain on the body. This level of activity also activates the parasympathetic nervous system post-exercise, which helps lower cortisol levels and supports recovery. Activities like brisk walking, swimming, or cycling for 30–45 minutes are accessible options that provide these benefits while being gentle enough to avoid overloading the body.

In contrast, high-intensity exercise—activities performed at 70–90% of your maximum heart rate—can temporarily increase cortisol levels as part of the body's natural response to physical stress. While this can be beneficial in small doses, promoting improved endurance and metabolic health, prolonged or frequent high-intensity exercise may lead to chronically elevated cortisol levels, especially in those of us already under significant stress or dealing with inadequate recovery. Over time, this can contribute to fatigue, impaired immune function, and heightened stress sensitivity.

For those who experience chronic stress, burnout, or conditions like adrenal fatigue, moderate-intensity exercise is generally preferable. It provides the benefits of movement and stress relief without exacerbating cortisol levels or depleting energy reserves. High-intensity workouts may still be beneficial but should be balanced with adequate rest. In cases of chronic stress, they can be included less frequently to prevent overtraining and additional strain on the mind and body.

EXERCISE AND MOVEMENT FOR STRESS REDUCTION

Selecting appropriate cardio activities will imply considering both your fitness level and cortisol management goals. Low-impact options like cycling and swimming are excellent choices, especially if you're looking to minimize joint strain while boosting cardiovascular health. These activities are gentle yet effective ways to maintain fitness and manage stress. For those who enjoy a bit more intensity, interval training with built-in rest periods can be highly effective. Alternating between bursts of activity and recovery allows you to challenge your body, improve fitness, and regulate cortisol levels. As always, the key is to listen to your body and choose exercises that align with your personal preferences and health objectives, ensuring that your routine is both enjoyable and sustainable.

Creating a routine that blends intensity with relaxation can truly help maintain this balance. Perhaps start your day with a brisk walk, followed by a series of gentle stretches. Alternatively, you could join a dance class that emphasizes fun and movement. Dance is one of the outlets that provides an opportunity to express yourself, engage with others, and enjoy a cardiovascular workout without the monotony of traditional exercises. The joy of moving to music reduces stress and enhances our mood, making it an ideal way to incorporate cardio into your life.

Let's talk about the unsung hero of fitness and stress management: rest and recovery. Yes, the part where you don't work out. Shocking, I know. But here's the deal—these aren't just bonus features you sprinkle in when you "have time." They are mission-critical for keeping your hormones happy and your cortisol levels from going full-blown disaster mode. Exercise naturally spikes cortisol (which is fine, it's doing its thing), but if you treat your workouts like an Olympic event every single day without giving your body a break, you're basically sending it an eviction notice. Chronic overtraining can leave you exhausted, wreck your immune system, and even start breaking down your hard-earned muscle.

So, if you needed permission to take that rest day? Consider this it. Rest days are the times when the real magic happens—your muscles rebuild stronger, your energy stores replenish, and your nervous system rebalances. But recovery isn't just about lying on the couch. Active recovery techniques like gentle yoga, leisurely walks, or light stretching can keep blood flowing, reduce muscle stiffness, and even help flush out metabolic waste from your workouts.

And then there's sleep, the essential yet often overlooked key to recovery. Inadequate sleep exacerbates cortisol spikes, leaving you feeling drained and irritable, which can derail both your fitness and stress-management goals. Quality sleep is when your body does its most profound healing work, from releasing growth hormone to repairing tissues and regulating cortisol levels. Aim for 7–9 hours of uninterrupted sleep per night, optimizing your environment with cool temperatures, minimal light, and a consistent bedtime routine. By prioritizing rest and recovery, you will prevent burnout while setting yourself up for sustainable progress, better energy, and a healthier relationship with exercise. It's a reminder that sometimes the most productive thing you can do is simply let your body rest.

Strength Training to Reduce Stress

STRENGTH TRAINING IS A HIGHLY effective way to build both physical strength and mental resilience. For those already familiar with exercise science, its role in managing cortisol is especially compelling. Resistance exercises, such as weightlifting or body-weight movements, challenge your muscles and enhance lean muscle growth, which is key to supporting metabolic efficiency.

As previously discussed, cortisol levels naturally rise during exercise, supporting the energy needed for physical exertion. However, regular strength training can improve your body's ability to regulate this hormone. Over time, consistent training leads to adaptations that lower baseline cortisol levels, reduce excessive stress responses, and enhance overall hormonal balance. This helps maintain a calmer state of mind and better recovery from daily stressors.

Additionally, strength training stimulates the release of endorphins, improves insulin sensitivity, and increases bone density, making it a cornerstone of long-term physical and mental health. For those balancing demanding schedules or high-stress environments, integrating resistance exercises into your routine will provide both immediate stress relief and sustainable benefits to your overall health.

Before engaging in strength training, it would be wise to be familiar with the principles of progressive overload. This means gradually increasing the resistance or difficulty of your exercises to continue challenging your muscles. It's like teaching your body to handle more, bit by bit, without overloading the system. Equally important is maintaining proper form and technique. This will ensure that you're working the intended muscles, while also reducing the risk of injury and unnecessary damage to joints and articulations. Imagine your spine aligned, your core engaged, and your movements controlled, each lift a mindful action, focused on the quality of the movement rather than the quantity. Effective strength training involves listening to your body, respecting its limits, and gradually pushing those boundaries.

For those just starting, bodyweight exercises provide an accessible entry point. Think of squats, push-ups, or planks—simple movements that can be done anywhere, requiring no equipment yet offering significant benefits. As you progress, experimenting with resistance bands or free weights can add variety and challenge. Resistance bands are versatile and gentle on the joints, while free weights allow for more dynamic movements. A sample routine might include a combination of squats, lunges, and overhead presses, tailored to fit your fitness level and preferences. These exercises engage multiple muscle groups, enhancing strength and coordination, all while maintaining a focus on proper form and safety.

Unfortunately, strength training often comes with misconceptions, particularly for women. Many worry about bulking up, fearing that lifting weights will lead to an overly muscular physique. The truth is, achieving significant muscle mass requires an intensive combination of high-volume training, calorie surplus, and precise macronutrient intake—conditions unlikely to result from a typical strength training routine. Instead, regular resistance exercises will help improve muscle tone, physical definition, and overall confidence.

More importantly, strength training plays a critical role in long-term bone health. Weight-bearing exercises, like squats, deadlifts, and resistance band workouts, stimulate osteoblast activity, which promotes the production of new bone tissue. Over time, this process increases bone density, lowering the risk of osteoporosis and fractures, particularly as we age. For women, whose bone density naturally declines after menopause, strength training can be a powerful tool to maintain skeletal integrity.

Strength training isn't just about looking good in your favorite jeans (though, let's be honest, that's a solid perk). It's about keeping your body strong, capable, and ready to handle whatever life throws at you, whether that's hauling groceries, wrangling toddlers, or opening that ridiculously stubborn pickle jar. Just two to three sessions a week can boost your strength, improve mobility, and set you up for long-term health. Plus, future you will thank you when you're effortlessly carrying all the shopping bags in one trip like the badass you are.

Stretching and Flexibility for Hormonal Health

STARTING your day with a stretch can feel like a small act, but it has meaningful impacts on your health. Stretching isn't just about flexibility, as it plays an essential role in stress management and hormonal balance. Research shows that regular stretching can help lower cortisol, which tends to spike during periods of physical or emotional tension. By engaging in even a few minutes of stretching, you can help your muscles relax, improve circulation, and support your body's natural stress-reduction mechanisms. Better blood flow also means more oxygen and nutrients are delivered to your tissues, enhancing recovery and promoting a sense of calm. For many, this simple, intentional practice becomes a cornerstone of maintaining physical readiness and emotional equilibrium, particularly in today's fast-paced environment.

There are various stretching techniques to choose from, each serving a specific purpose. Static stretching involves holding a position for an extended period, usually 15 to 60 seconds. This method is excellent for relaxation and post-exercise cool-downs, as it helps increase muscle length and joint flexibility. Dynamic stretching, on the other hand, consists of moving parts of your body through a full range of motion, such as arm circles or leg swings. It's ideal for warming up before physical activity, as it prepares your muscles for exertion while maintaining flexibility. Proprioceptive Neuromuscular Facilitation, or PNF stretching, combines passive stretching and isometric contractions. Though more advanced, PNF is effective in enhancing flexibility and strength simultaneously. Understanding these techniques will allow you to choose the most suitable for your needs, enriching your routine with versatility and depth.

Creating a stretching sequence tailored for hormonal health focuses on areas most affected by hormonal shifts. Hip-opening stretches, such as the butterfly pose or lunges, can release tension stored in the pelvis and lower back, regions often impacted by hormonal changes. These stretches encourage the flow of energy and promote relaxation, making them particularly beneficial during times of hormonal fluctuation. Gentle backbends, like the cat-cow stretch, provide relief from stress by opening the chest and elon-

THE COMPLETE CORTISOL DETOX HANDBOOK

gating the spine. These movements both ease physical tension and invite emotional release.

Putting in place a daily stretching routine is both practical and rewarding. A morning stretch sequence, perhaps as simple as reaching for the sky or rolling your shoulders, can set a positive, grounded, and energized tone for the day. These moments of intentional movement gently wake up your body, preparing you mentally and physically for the tasks ahead. Throughout the day, especially if you find yourself mostly seated, desk stretches become invaluable. Taking a few minutes to move your arms, neck, and back can refresh your mind and relieve the physical strain of prolonged sitting. These small breaks will improve your posture, help prevent repetitive strain injuries, and re-energize your focus.

Creating an Exercise Routine That Sticks

STICKING to an exercise routine in the chaos of everyday life takes more than just good intentions; it requires strategy (and maybe a little bribery in the form of post-workout snacks). Start by setting fitness goals that won't make you want to fake an injury. If you tell yourself you'll run 10 miles a day when you currently get winded walking to the fridge, you're setting yourself up for disappointment. Instead, aim for something manageable, like a 30-minute daily walk or a couple of yoga sessions each week. The goal is to feel accomplished, not like you've signed up for a boot camp you can't escape.

Next, pick a workout time that actually fits your life. If you're not a morning person, don't convince yourself you'll be up at 5 a.m. doing squats—you won't. Find a time that works, whether it's post-dinner, lunch break, or whenever your favorite show is on (hello, treadmill entertainment). The key is consistency. Make exercise a non-negotiable part of your day, like brushing your teeth or waiting in line for your (single) daily coffee. Once it becomes part of your routine, it won't feel like a chore—it'll just be what you do.

Variety is the ingredient that will help keep the spark alive in your routine, preventing it from becoming tedious. You may want to include different types of workouts to keep things fresh and engaging. Rotate between cardio, strength, flexibility, and mindful movement activities throughout the week. One day might involve a brisk outdoor walk, while another could see you engaging in a Pilates session. This diversity works different muscle groups while keeping your mind engaged. Seasonal activities should also be considered. In the warmer months, swimming or hiking might be appealing, while colder weather could usher in indoor cycling or dance classes. These shifts ensure that exercise remains enjoyable, adapting to both your environment and your interests. Again, when workouts feel like play rather than work, motivation naturally follows.

Sticking to an exercise routine can come with its own set of challenges. Motivation can wane, especially when life gets hectic. Combat this by setting up a reward system, where you treat yourself for meeting your fitness goals. Rewards can be as simple as a relaxing bath, a new book, a spa treatment or a favorite show. If time constraints are another hurdle, break workouts into smaller chunks throughout the day. If a full session feels daunting, you might find that ten-minute intervals can accumulate into a substantial workout by day's end. Remember, flexibility in your schedule doesn't imply inconsistency. Self-care means doing what works best for *you*. Strive to adjust your routine to fit the ebb and flow of life while maintaining your commitment to movement.

Leveraging tracking tools and support systems can further cement your exercise habits. Fitness apps offer a convenient way to log workouts, track progress, and set reminders, turning your phone into a personal coach. These apps often provide insights into your activity patterns, which can help identify areas for improvement. Joining local or online workout groups can also add a social dimension to your fitness journey. Being part of a community boosts accountability and provides encouragement. Whether it's a running club or a virtual fitness class, connecting with others who share similar goals can make exercise feel like a shared adventure rather than a solitary task.

Finally, the key with exercise lies in crafting a plan that resonates with you—one that adapts to life's changes yet remains steadfast in its pursuit of health. As you continue to explore the transformative power of movement, keep in mind that each step, stretch, and lift brings you closer to balance and vitality.

FIVE
STRESS MANAGEMENT AND EMOTIONAL RESILIENCE

WE'VE all had those moments—your inbox is overflowing, your phone won't stop buzzing, and the to-do list feels endless. It's like your brain is hosting a never-ending meeting where everyone is shouting over each other. Sound familiar? That's where mindfulness and meditation come in, not as magic fixes but as scientifically-backed tools to help you regain a sense of control and calm.

Think of it like this: Instead of doom-scrolling social media at the end of a long day, you could spend 10 minutes meditating and actually feel better afterward. Or try mindfulness while eating, savoring that first sip of coffee instead of guzzling it in three gulps while running out the door. These practices aren't about escaping reality, but rather about learning to navigate it with a bit more grace (and a lot less stress). Let's face it, we could all use that.

Mindfulness itself is a concept of presence, of being fully engaged in the moment you're living, rather than being consumed by thoughts of the past or worries about the future. It's the art of paying attention to your surroundings, your emotions, and your bodily sensations without judgment. Meditation, on the other hand, is like the anchor that steadies the ship; it guides the mind into stillness and clarity. Together, they form a powerful duo in stress reduction. Research such as the Shamatha Project at the University of California has shown that mindfulness achieved through meditation is, in fact, associated with lower levels of cortisol. It promotes emotional balance by reducing the tendency to ruminate, which often triggers cortisol release.

However, the benefits of regular mindfulness and meditation extend far beyond momentary relaxation. These practices can significantly reduce symptoms of anxiety, allowing us to navigate life's challenges with greater ease. By cultivating a state of calm awareness, we enhance our emotional regulation, responding to stress with composure rather than reaction. This clarity of mind helps in stressful situations and permeates our daily lives, offering a lens of tranquillity through which to view our surroundings. Over time, consistent practice creates changes in our mental landscape, leading to a sense of peace and resilience that becomes second nature.

Starting a mindfulness practice might seem daunting, but it begins with small, intentional steps. Dedicate a specific time each day to practice; even five minutes can make a difference. To ease into mindfulness, I highly recommend exploring the world of guided meditation apps. These digital companions offer structured sessions to gently lead you through your practice. These tools can be invaluable, especially for beginners who may feel unsure about where to start. As you progress, you'll find it easier to extend your practice, allowing it to naturally integrate into your daily routine through unprompted mindful moments. The key is consistency, making it a regular part of your life rather than an occasional escape.

A popular method of adding these practices to daily life is with something as straightforward as a body scan meditation. Start by finding a comfortable position, either seated or lying down. Closing your eyes, gently shifting your attention through your body, starting from your head down to your toes. Pay attention to each part of the

STRESS MANAGEMENT AND EMOTIONAL RESILIENCE

body, noticing any sensations, areas of tension, or relaxation, without attempting to alter them. This involves lying down or sitting comfortably, closing your eyes, and bringing awareness to each part of your body in turn, from the top of your head to the tips of your toes. Notice any sensations, tensions, or areas of relaxation without trying to change them.

Another fun and beneficial exercise is mindful walking. As you walk, focus on the sensation of your feet touching the ground, the rhythm of your breath, and the sounds around you. This practice transforms an everyday activity into a grounding experience, connecting you with the present moment.

Mindfulness Reflection Prompts

Set aside a few minutes each day to journal about your mindfulness practice. In a quiet, distraction-free space, reflect on how it feels to be present, any challenges you encounter, and the impact on your stress levels.

1. Morning Intention Setting

- What do I want to focus on today to bring myself a sense of calm and clarity?
- How can I remind myself to stay present and mindful throughout the day?

2. Midday Check-In

- What emotions have surfaced so far today, and how have I responded to them?
- Is there anything causing tension or stress right now? How can I approach it mindfully?

3. Evening Reflection

- What moments today made me feel centered or connected to myself?
- Were there times I acted reactively? What could I do differently next time?

4. Gratitude and Growth

- What am I grateful for today, and how has it influenced my emotional state?

- What is one small step I can take tomorrow to enhance my mindfulness practice?

PRO TIP: *Pair this journaling practice with a calming ritual like deep breathing, a warm cup of herbal tea, or soft instrumental music to create a nurturing environment.*

Breathing Techniques for Instant Stress Relief

We've all faced those tense moments where our heart races like it's trying to set a new record, and our stress levels could power a small city. In times like these, it's easy to feel at the mercy of our body's fight-or-flight response. But here's the good news: we already have a built-in tool to take back control: our breath.

Breathing is the essence of life and a direct line to our nervous system. By practicing conscious breathing techniques, we can activate our parasympathetic nervous system, the "rest-and-digest" counterpart to the adrenaline-fueled fight-or-flight mode. This simple shift helps lower heart rate, reduce blood pressure, and brings clarity to our frazzled mind. For example, box breathing—inhale for four counts, hold for four, exhale for four, and pause for four—can be done discreetly at your desk while everyone else is stressing over the latest deadline. It's a stress relief hack, minus the need for expensive gadgets or apps.

Breathing techniques are diverse and adaptable, all of them offering immediate relief from stress. Diaphragmatic breathing, often called belly breathing, is a cornerstone practice. It involves inhaling deeply through the nose, allowing your belly to rise as your diaphragm expands. This technique increases oxygen exchange and promotes relaxation. Another effective method is the 4-7-8 breathing technique, which acts as a reset button for your stress response. To practice, sit comfortably, inhale through your nose for four counts, hold for seven, and then exhale through your mouth for eight counts. This rhythmic breathing pattern helps regulate cortisol levels and calms the mind and body.

To experience the full benefits of these techniques, proper practice is key. Start by finding a comfortable position—whether seated or lying down—where you can relax without distractions. Close your eyes if you wish, and focus on your breath. As you inhale deeply, feel your abdomen rise, and as you exhale, notice it gently fall. With the 4-7-8 method, focus on the count, letting it guide your breath. Although these exercises are rooted in the body, they will engage your mind, drawing attention away from stress and into the soothing rhythm of your breath. With regular practice, these techniques will become instinctive, ready to support you whenever stress arises.

An important benefit of breath work is the versatility of practices. In the midst of a stressful meeting, you can discreetly employ diaphragmatic breathing, letting the tension melt away with each breath. Before sleep, the 4-7-8 method can act as a lullaby for your mind, easing you into restful slumber. The beauty of these practices lies in their adaptability to your needs, whether you're navigating a hectic day or seeking peace at bedtime. They can empower you to take control, offering a pocket-sized tool for stress relief that is always within reach.

Stress-Busting Breathing Cards

This is a collection of small, card-style instructions for various breathing techniques. Each card can be copied in your journal or saved digitally, making them easily accessible as quick reminders during your day.

Card 1: 4-7-8 Breathing

PURPOSE: Calm your mind and body quickly.

1. Inhale deeply through your nose for 4 seconds.
2. Hold your breath for 7 seconds.
3. Exhale slowly through your mouth for 8 seconds.
4. Repeat 4 times.

Card 2: Box Breathing

PURPOSE: Center yourself and reduce stress.

1. Inhale through your nose for 4 seconds.
2. Hold your breath for 4 seconds.
3. Exhale through your mouth for 4 seconds.
4. Hold your breath again for 4 seconds.
5. Repeat the cycle 4 times.

Card 3: Alternate Nostril Breathing

PURPOSE: Balance your energy and reduce anxiety.

STRESS MANAGEMENT AND EMOTIONAL RESILIENCE

1. Close your right nostril with your thumb.
2. Inhale deeply through your left nostril for 4 seconds.
3. Close your left nostril with your ring finger, releasing your thumb from the right nostril.
4. Exhale through your right nostril for 4 seconds.
5. Repeat on the other side. Continue for 2 minutes.

Card 4: Diaphragmatic Breathing

PURPOSE: Activate your body's relaxation response.

1. Place one hand on your chest and the other on your belly.
2. Inhale deeply through your nose, feeling your belly rise (not your chest).
3. Exhale slowly through your mouth, feeling your belly fall.
4. Continue for 3-5 minutes.

Card 5: Ocean Breath (Ujjayi)

PURPOSE: Soothe your nervous system.

1. Inhale deeply through your nose, slightly constricting the back of your throat.
2. Exhale through your nose with the same throat constriction, creating a soft "ocean wave" sound.
3. Maintain a steady rhythm for 2-3 minutes.

Card 6: 5-5-5 Breathing

PURPOSE: Reset your focus during stressful moments.

1. Inhale through your nose for 5 seconds.
2. Hold your breath for 5 seconds.
3. Exhale through your mouth for 5 seconds.
4. Repeat as needed until you feel grounded.

Card 7: Humming Bee Breath (Bhramari)

PURPOSE: Quiet the mind and reduce tension.

1. Close your eyes and take a deep breath in through your nose.
2. As you exhale, hum softly like a bee, focusing on the vibration.
3. Continue for 5 breaths.

Card 8: Simple 3-Step Reset

PURPOSE: Quick stress relief in under a minute.

1. Inhale through your nose for 3 seconds.
2. Exhale through your mouth for 6 seconds.
3. Pause for 3 seconds before repeating.
4. Do this for 3 rounds.

STRESS MANAGEMENT AND EMOTIONAL RESILIENCE

Tips for Use:

- Keep these cards in your purse, on your desk, or saved on your phone for quick access.
- Use them during moments of stress, or as part of your daily routine to manage cortisol levels effectively.

Building Emotional Resilience: Handling Life's Curveballs

LIFE OFTEN FEELS like a series of unexpected twists and turns, testing our ability to adapt and persevere. Emotional resilience is our capacity to bounce back from these challenges. It is the inner strength that keeps us steady when faced with adversity. Resilience isn't about avoiding difficulties, but about meeting them head-on, learning, and growing stronger. In the long term, building resilience supports mental health, acting as a buffer against stress and anxiety. It empowers us to navigate life's ups and downs with confidence, turning setbacks into stepping stones toward personal growth.

Cultivating resilience involves so much more than having a positive outlook—it's about grounding ourselves in strategies that actually work. A growth mindset, for example, shifts our focus from "I can't" to "How can I?" Research by Dr. Carol Dweck has shown that believing in your capacity to improve through effort can significantly enhance problem-solving and performance. Think of it like learning to cook a new dish. You might burn it the first few times, but with practice (and maybe a call to your mom or a Google search), you get better. The same principle applies to tackling life's bigger challenges.

Equally, if not more important, is building strong social connections. Humans are hardwired for connection, and research confirms that meaningful relationships directly impact mental and physical health. Engaging with supportive people activates our parasympathetic nervous system, creating a state of calm and safety. Essentially, our body responds to social warmth by dialing down stress hormones like cortisol and boosting feel-good chemicals like oxytocin. That's why venting to a friend over coffee or sharing a laugh during game night feels so good—it's science at work.

These connections also help regulate our physiological state by mitigating our body's threat response. When you face stress alone, your brain's amygdala sounds the alarm, flooding your system with stress hormones. But talking through your worries with someone you trust can signal to your brain that you're safe, quieting the alarm bells.

Let's be real: life is messy. From dealing with demanding bosses to toddlers refusing to eat anything but crackers, stress is unavoidable. But having people in your corner, whether it's a friend who can turn your rant into a laugh or a partner who reminds you to breathe, makes the chaos more manageable. Resilience grows not just from internal strength but also from leaning on and supporting others.

Many resilience development practices can easily be added to any routine. Journaling is a powerful tool for self-reflection, one that allows us to process emotions and gain clarity in difficult situations. By putting thoughts on paper, we create a safe space to explore feelings and devise strategies for moving forward. Additionally, setting realistic goals and expectations helps maintain focus and motivation. Break larger tasks into manageable steps, celebrating small victories along the way. This approach reduces overwhelm and builds momentum, reinforcing your ability to tackle challenges effectively.

Work-Life Balance: Managing Stress in a Busy World

Balancing the demands of work and personal life can often feel like walking a tightrope, where any misstep might send everything tumbling. The pressure from workplace demands is relentless, sometimes requiring us to be available around the clock, whether it's dealing with emails that never seem to stop or meeting deadlines that loom like dark clouds. This constant hustle can bleed into personal time, leaving little room for relaxation or family. At home, family obligations call for attention, demanding energy and patience. Whether it's helping with homework, managing household chores, or nurturing relationships, the list of responsibilities seems never-ending. These competing demands often lead to a feeling of being stretched too thin, where both work and family life suffer, creating a cycle of stress that is hard to break.

Bringing balance to your life isn't some mystical, unattainable goal; it requires a bit of strategy and a good dose of intentionality. One tool that really works is the Eisenhower Box. This simple matrix helps categorize tasks by urgency and importance, essentially forcing us to focus on what actually matters. It's like having a filter for all those endless to-dos. There are the "urgent and important" tasks (which are the ones you focus on first), and then the "not urgent but important" tasks (these are where you want to put in some real thought and planning). Then, there's the "urgent but not important" stuff (like answering that email about a meeting next month that could've been handled by someone else). Finally, "not urgent and not important" items are comprised of things that drain energy without actually adding value (so let it go). Trust me, once you've separated these, the chaos of daily life feels a lot more manageable.

Setting boundaries is just as crucial, if not more so. Make sure your work and personal life don't start overlapping. It's important to set clear limits, like defining specific work hours and resisting the urge to check your email when you're supposed to be unwinding. It's not easy (especially when your boss thinks emails should be answered at 11 p.m. on a Friday), but if you communicate your boundaries to your employer and colleagues, you will create an environment where respect is mutual. It helps everyone stay on the same page and, quite frankly, it gives you the mental space to recharge without feeling like you're always on call. Science backs this up, too: studies have shown that maintaining boundaries reduces burnout and helps sustain focus, which in turn boosts productivity and overall well-being. You don't have to do everything, you just have to do the right things—and that's where the balance lies.

Self-care is another essential component of stress management. It isn't just some luxury you can squeeze in when you have time,

STRESS MANAGEMENT AND EMOTIONAL RESILIENCE

but rather is at the heart of staying mentally and emotionally healthy. Regular "me time" is necessary for recharging. Activities like taking short breaks, walking in nature, or engaging in hobbies lowers cortisol levels and reduces stress.

Even if it's just ten minutes to yourself, it counts. I'm talking about those quiet moments with a book, a brisk walk, or doing something that genuinely brings you joy (yes, even if it's just Instagram for a minute). Sometimes it's hard to find time, especially with all the tasks piling up. But the more you prioritize these moments, the better you will be able to handle stress and stay on top of your game.

Finally, let's talk about effective communication, another key component for maintaining balance in life. Everyone benefits from being clear and honest about their needs and boundaries, whether at work or at home. Research consistently shows that setting boundaries helps reduce stress and increase job satisfaction. For example, talking to your employer about flexible work options like remote work or adjusting hours can actually improve productivity and job performance.

At home, communication is just as important. It's easy to fall into the trap of doing everything yourself (especially if you're a chronic overachiever), but sharing household responsibilities can make a huge difference. In fact, when tasks are divided fairly, stress levels drop and family bonds strengthen. It might feel like a small win when everyone finally pitches in to clean up after dinner, but it actually improves overall relationship satisfaction, creating a supportive environment where no one feels like they're carrying the whole load. So, whether it's scheduling your workday or divvying up chores, clear and open communication leads to a more balanced life where work and personal time complement each other rather than compete.

These simple things to begin implementing in your life will give your brain and body a chance to reset, which can make a huge difference when it comes to preventing burnout. Think of it as hitting your reset button. When you give yourself a moment to breathe, organize your priorities, speak your mind and recharge, you're building resilience. Plus, it's a nice reminder that you're human, not a productivity robot.

Digital Detox: Reducing Stress from Technology

THINK ABOUT A TYPICAL DAY: you wake up to the blue glow of your phone, sifting through notifications before you've even sat up. From there, it's a non-stop stream—work emails, texts, Messenger pings, social media scrolls, and maybe a few too many reminders to "update your software." By the time you're supposed to relax, you're still glued to a screen, whether it's Netflix, TikTok, or doomscrolling the news.

The constant connectivity feels productive but often has the opposite effect. In fact, studies show that excessive screen time increases cortisol levels. Your brain isn't designed to process this much information at once, and that overload leads to decision fatigue. Each ping interrupts your focus, with research indicating it can take up to 23 minutes to fully refocus after a distraction. Now multiply that by the dozens of notifications you get daily.

This constant engagement doesn't just disrupt your workflow; it erodes the line between work and personal time. The boundaries between work and personal life blur as technology follows you home, making it difficult to truly disconnect and relax. Responding to a work email late at night might feel responsible, but it's also a fast track to burnout. Your brain stays in a heightened state of alertness, unable to fully disengage and recharge. And, as we know, chronic exposure to this stress cycle is linked to anxiety, poor sleep quality, and even a weakened immune system.

We all know it's a problem; yet, when your phone suggests "screen time is up 15% this week," the best you can manage is an eye roll. The good news? Small, intentional changes, like setting

STRESS MANAGEMENT AND EMOTIONAL RESILIENCE

app limits or carving out phone-free time, can help break the cycle and give your brain the breather it desperately needs.

The concept of a digital detox offers a refreshing counterbalance to this digital deluge. This is the act of stepping back from screens to reconnect with the tangible world around you. By intentionally reducing screen time, you create space to engage with offline activities that nourish your soul and calm your mind. The potential benefits are significant: stress levels decrease, your capacity for deep thinking improves, and you rediscover the joy of simple pleasures. This doesn't mean abandoning technology altogether, but rather setting boundaries that allow you to regain control over your time and attention. A digital detox isn't about deprivation. Instead, it gives us some much-needed perspective to make more conscious choices that enhance your quality of life.

Implementing a digital detox can feel surprisingly refreshing, and it doesn't require drastic measures, just intentional steps. You can start by scheduling specific times during the day to step away from screens. For instance, designate the first hour after waking up as tech-free. Instead of scrolling through your phone, enjoy a distraction-free breakfast or a quick walk to clear your mind. In the evening, trade binge-watching for a good book or some light stretching, a win for your eyes and your brain.

Creating a tech-free bedroom is another game-changer. Exposure to blue light from screens disrupts melatonin production, making it harder to fall asleep. Removing devices from your sleeping space will therefore help improve sleep quality and reinforces your bedroom as a place for rest, not scrolling or email-checking marathons. To make the switch easier, you can get an old-school alarm clock. Sure, it doesn't let you check your socials, but that's the point. Plus, there's something very satisfying about slapping a physical snooze button.

If the idea of giving up screen time feels daunting, remember that even small steps help. Take breaks during the day. Leave your phone behind while running errands or use airplane mode during dinner. You might quickly notice how life without constant notifications is less stressful and more productive.

As you reduce your screen time, explore alternative activities that invite relaxation and creativity. One option is to dive into the pages of a physical book, savoring the tactile experience and the opportunity to immerse yourself in a different world. Reading stimulates the mind and offers a peaceful escape from the constant buzz of digital information. Otherwise, pursuing creative hobbies like painting, playing a musical instrument, or crafting are excellent options. These activities engage different parts of the brain, creating a sense of accomplishment and joy. They encourage us to express ourselves in ways that screens cannot, grounding us in the present moment and allowing stress to melt away.

The Power of Positive Thinking: Mental Detox Strategies

OVER TIME, our minds can become cluttered with patterns of negative thinking, much like an overflowing email inbox filled with spam. You know the ones—unnecessary self-criticisms that pop up at the worst times, like "You're not good enough" or "You'll never figure this out". Left unchecked, these thoughts tend to drain our mental energy and affect our overall well-being.

A mental detox doesn't imply ignoring these thoughts; it's about recognizing and actively challenging them. Repetitive negative thinking is linked to higher stress levels and even physical health issues like increased inflammation. Reframing these thoughts, such as viewing mistakes as learning opportunities rather than failures, can help build resilience and emotional balance. For example, instead of berating yourself for sending an email with a typo, remind yourself it happens to everyone.

Now, building a positive mindset requires more than just "thinking happy thoughts." It involves practices like journaling to

STRESS MANAGEMENT AND EMOTIONAL RESILIENCE

identify thought patterns, mindfulness to stay present, and even gratitude exercises, which studies show can boost serotonin and dopamine levels. It might feel awkward at first, writing down that you're grateful for your coffee machine's ability to save your mornings, but these small actions will rewire your brain over time. Think of this process as mental hygiene: less glamorous than a spa day but far more impactful. By addressing negativity head-on, you will clear space for confidence and happiness while setting yourself up to handle life's inevitable chaos with a little more humor and grace.

So, let's look at some practical mind-detox strategies.

To boost your mental well-being, try starting a gratitude journaling practice as part of your daily routine. Set aside time each day to reflect on what you're thankful for, no matter how small. Recording these moments will help you focus on the positive aspects of your life, enhancing your overall mood and outlook. Additionally, using affirmations can reinforce your self-empowerment. These are positive statements that increase your strengths and potential, helping to silence the inner critic. By repeating affirmations regularly, you will build a foundation of self-belief and optimism, transforming your internal dialogue into one of encouragement and support.

Positive thinking exercises can also play a role in mental detoxification. Reframing negative thoughts is one such exercise, where you consciously challenge and alter pessimistic views. For example, if you catch yourself thinking, "I'll never succeed at this," reframe it to, "I have the skills to learn and improve." This practice will shift your mindset and build resilience as you learn to approach challenges with a constructive attitude.

Visualization is another practical and evidence-based technique for improving focus and motivation. Mentally rehearsing positive outcomes activates the same neural pathways involved in actual performance, helping to prime your brain for success. For example, athletes often use visualization to prepare for competitions, mentally practicing their routines or envisioning crossing the finish line. This isn't wishful thinking, but intentionally training your brain to recognize opportunities and make better decisions.

To begin, think of a goal you're working toward, whether it's nailing a presentation, hitting a fitness milestone, or finally tackling that overstuffed email inbox. Spend a few minutes each day visualizing yourself succeeding: delivering your speech confidently, feeling strong after your workout, or seeing an empty inbox and a coffee in hand to celebrate. This exercise will help clarify your goals while reducing anxiety by making the process feel familiar.

And don't worry—this is not about pretending everything will magically fall into place. Visualization works best when paired with action. After all, no amount of mental rehearsal will empty the dishwasher or write that report for you (if only). However, mental rehearsal activates the same neural pathways in the brain as actual practice, which helps build the skills and confidence needed to perform tasks effectively.

In everyday life, visualization can help you stay focused and motivated. Say you're dreading a big work presentation. Instead of spiraling into stress, take a few minutes to visualize yourself delivering it confidently, hitting all the key points, and fielding questions with ease. This primes your brain to approach the task with a positive mindset, increasing the likelihood of success. And yes, this applies to the small stuff too. Visualizing an organized home might just give you the nudge to tackle that overflowing laundry basket.

The key here is consistency. Regularly visualizing what success looks like can train your brain to focus on the steps needed to achieve it. Just don't get stuck daydreaming, as no amount of mental rehearsal will hit "submit" on your tax return or meal-prep your week's lunches (if only neuroscience could handle chores). Pairing visualization with deliberate action creates a powerful combination, which will help you turn aspirations into achievements.

Next, creating a positive environment around you is an essential part of supporting a mental detox. Our surroundings and social interactions have a huge impact on our mental health. For example, having supportive friends and engaging with media that fosters growth and positivity can actually help lower cortisol levels and promote the release of dopamine. That's why spending time with people who encourage your goals or reading material that challenges you to grow is key. It gives your brain a break from the constant barrage of negativity.

Let's take a moment to talk about clutter, both the kind taking over your countertops and the kind clogging up your brain. A messy space isn't just an eyesore, it's a certified stress booster, making it harder to focus and zapping productivity. Ever tried to work while surrounded by half-finished projects, unopened mail, and that "one day" pile of fitness magazines? It's like trying to meditate in the middle of a rock concert. Clearing out the unnecessary, whether it's expired coupons, mystery Tupperware lids, or mental baggage from that awkward email you sent two years ago, creates space for actual peace of mind. No, this isn't me pushing you to become a minimalist guru who owns one chair and a houseplant. It's just a friendly nudge to ditch the excess so your brain can finally breathe.

And here's the thing: cultivating a positive space doesn't mean ignoring the tough stuff. Life's challenges are real, but when you've cleared mental clutter and surrounded yourself with positivity, you're better equipped to tackle them head-on. You are setting your brain up with the mental equivalent of a solid gym routine, strengthening your mindset to deal with whatever comes your way.

In the next section, we'll dive deeper into how you can build these habits into your everyday life, making them second nature so you can thrive in the long term. And yes, it is absolutely possible to get there without turning your home into a shrine of Zen.

SIX
LIFESTYLE CHANGES FOR LONG-TERM BALANCE

IN A WORLD that never seems to slow down, finding balance can feel like an elusive dream. You may often find yourself juggling multiple roles and responsibilities, with little time left to catch your breath. But what if I told you that one of the most powerful tools for maintaining equilibrium in life is something as simple as sleep? It could be as easy as waking up each morning, refreshed and ready to embrace the day, without the grogginess that accompanies most restless nights. Sleep may appear to be a passive state, but it is in fact an active process that plays a crucial role in regulating hormones, including cortisol. Quality sleep is your body's natural antidote to stress, helping to keep stress hormone levels in check and allowing you to face each day with clarity and calm.

Sleep acts as a reset button for the body's internal systems. It keeps your body and mind running smoothly. During deep sleep (slow-wave sleep), your body releases growth hormone, which is vital for repairing tissues, building muscle, and even keeping your skin looking its best. At night, melatonin takes center stage, helping you fall asleep and stay asleep while keeping your circadian rhythms in check. It's your body's internal clock whispering, "Hey, it's time to wind down."

Cortisol, in contrast, follows a natural pattern, rising in the early morning to prepare you for the day ahead. When sleep is disrupted, these rhythms become misaligned, leading to an array of health issues. Sleep deprivation can elevate cortisol levels, contributing to feelings of stress and anxiety. Over time, this can increase your risk of obesity and diabetes, as poor sleep affects glucose metabolism and insulin sensitivity.

Therefore, ensuring plentiful quality sleep should be a health priority. To improve your sleep, first focus on creating an environment that aligns with your body's natural sleep-wake cycle. Start with temperature: research shows the ideal range for sleep is 60-67°F (15-19°C). If you're sweating through the night or bundling up like it's an Arctic expedition, your body won't relax enough to enter deeper sleep stages. Adjust your thermostat or switch to breathable bedding.

Lighting is another major player. Exposure to light at night suppresses melatonin, the hormone that signals it's time to sleep. Invest in blackout curtains or wear an eye mask that doesn't make you feel like a superhero in training. If your partner insists on late-night TikTok marathons, perhaps kindly remind them that even dim phone screens can disrupt circadian rhythms. And if you're in a noisy neighborhood or have a snoring pet (or partner), a white noise machine can work wonders by drowning out interruptions with soothing, consistent sound.

It is also worth considering making your bedroom a sleep-only zone. That means no scrolling through social media, no work emails, and definitely no late-night crime documentaries. Your brain needs a clear cue: the bed is for sleep (and, well, maybe one other thing). When your environment supports relaxation, your body immediately gets the message. You'll soon find yourself better rested, sharper, and maybe even less likely to snap when the coffee line takes an extra five minutes.

To further enhance your sleep quality, you can also establish a calming bedtime routine that transitions your mind and body from the busyness of the day to the tranquility of night. Gentle stretching or yoga can be incredibly effective in releasing physical tension and calming the mind. These activities encourage mindfulness and will help you tune into your body's needs. Alternatively, try trading screen time for a calming book, allowing the narrative to gently shift your focus away from daily stressors.

Maintain a consistent sleep schedule by setting a regular bedtime and wake-up time—even on weekends. Yes, that means resisting the urge to sabotage your progress for the sake of "just one more episode." Your circadian rhythm thrives on routine, and when you respect it, your body responds by making mornings far less punishing.

Finally, late-night eating is another culprit that can undermine quality sleep. Consuming heavy or rich foods too close to bedtime forces your digestive system to work overtime when it should be winding down. This can lead to discomfort, acid reflux, and fragmented sleep—not exactly a recipe for waking up refreshed. Late-night snacking also impacts melatonin production, especially if your go-to midnight indulgence includes sugar or processed carbs. And caffeine? If you're still sipping an espresso at 4 p.m., don't be surprised when your brain decides to host an impromptu TED Talk at 2 a.m.

Sticking to even a few of these simple strategies will help you wake up feeling rested, rather than wondering if quality sleep is just a myth.

Creating a Sleep Diary

Your sleep habits have a significant impact on cortisol levels and overall health. A sleep diary is a simple yet powerful tool to help you track your sleep patterns, identify disruptions, and uncover habits that may be interfering with restful sleep. Follow the steps below to start your personalized sleep diary journey.

Step 1: Choose Your Format
Decide how you want to track your sleep. Options include:

- **Digital:** Use an app or a spreadsheet.
- **Paper:** A notebook or printable template works well.

Step 2: What to Track
Include these key details in your diary:

- **Bedtime:** When did you go to bed?
- **Wake Time:** When did you wake up?
- **Sleep Duration:** How many hours did you sleep?
- **Sleep Quality:** Rate your sleep on a scale from 1 to 5.
- **Middle-of-the-Night Waking:** How often did you wake up, and for how long?
- **Pre-Sleep Routine:** What activities did you do before bed (e.g., reading, screen time)?
- **Mood:** How did you feel upon waking (e.g., refreshed, groggy)?

Step 3: Analyze Your Patterns

After a week, review your entries. Look for trends:

- Are late nights affecting your sleep quality?
- Is screen time before bed reducing your restfulness?
- Do consistent wake times improve your mood?

Tips for Success:

- Spend 2–3 minutes filling out your sleep diary every night before bed and jot down your wake-up details in the morning.
- Be consistent, even on weekends, to see accurate trends.
- Use the patterns you uncover to tweak your bedtime habits for better sleep and lower cortisol levels.

Crafting a Self-Care Routine: Prioritizing You

SELF-CARE ISN'T some frivolous luxury. In fact, just like putting on your own oxygen mask before helping anyone else, it's a survival strategy. And sure, bubble baths and spa days are nice (who doesn't love a good eucalyptus-scented escape?), but real self-care means consistently prioritizing your well-being so you don't crash and burn. Chronic stress without proper recovery isn't just exhausting; it can send your cortisol levels skyrocketing, wreck your sleep, weaken your immune system, and even set the stage for long-term health issues like hypertension and diabetes. In other words, skipping self-care isn't just a bad idea—it's practically an invitation for trouble.

Many of us, particularly women juggling work, family, and endless to-do lists, put ourselves last. You might recognize the pattern: skipping lunch to meet a deadline, saying yes to every favor until you're running on fumes, or convincing yourself you'll "relax later." Spoiler alert: "later" rarely comes unless you make it a priority. Regular self-assessment, such as asking yourself simple questions like "How am I feeling today?" or "What do I need right now?" is a practical starting point. Ignoring early signs of stress is like ignoring that gas light on your car. You might keep going for a while, but eventually, you *will* stall.

A personalized self-care plan doesn't have to be complicated. The goal is to find what works for you. If going to the gym feels like a chore, don't force it. Try a dance class instead, or even a brisk walk with your favorite podcast. If meditation feels like an Olympic event for your overthinking brain, that's okay; mindful activities like journaling or cooking can have similar benefits. Need a quick mood boost? Science suggests even a 10-minute walk in nature can reduce stress and improve focus. Pro tip: dogs make excellent accountability partners for this.

Humor can be part of self-care too. By lowering cortisol, laughter helps restore hormonal balance and promotes a sense of well-being. It also boosts endorphins, our body's natural feel-good chemicals, enhancing mood and reducing physical pain. So yes, watching that ridiculous sitcom or sharing memes with your best friend counts as self-care. It's a lighthearted way to nurture both your mind and your hormonal health.

Finally, let's (once more) address boundaries. Saying no doesn't make you a bad person; it makes you a smart one. Setting boundaries is crucial in protecting your self-care time. This involves learning to say no to non-essential obligations that drain your energy. Communicate your limits to friends and family, expressing the importance of this time for your well-being. This is not a selfish act, but rather ensures that you have the capacity to give your best in other areas of life. Prioritizing self-care might mean declining an invitation or delegating tasks, but it's a necessary step in maintaining your health. By managing commitments wisely, you will carve out essential space for self-care, recognizing its pivotal role in your health.

The Impact of Community and Support Systems

Amid the whirlwind of daily struggles, a strong support system isn't just nice to have. It is most essential, perhaps like coffee on a Monday morning or Wi-Fi that actually works. Social connections act as a built-in stress buffer, helping to regulate cortisol levels by providing both emotional reassurance and practical backup (because sometimes, you just need someone to remind you that no, you're not actually failing at life). The right people in your corner can turn overwhelming days into manageable ones and amplify the good moments with well-earned celebrations.

Building and nurturing these relationships takes time and effort, but the rewards are immense. Consider joining local clubs or interest groups where you can meet like-minded individuals who share your passions. Whether it's a book club, a gardening group, or a fitness class, these settings provide fertile ground for meaningful connections. Volunteering for community projects is another excellent way to foster relationships while making a positive impact. As you work alongside others toward a common goal, bonds naturally form, creating a network of support that can enhance your well-being. These relationships become a central aspect of your support system, offering strength and stability when you need it most.

Shared activities also play an important role in enhancing mental and emotional well-being. Participating in group exercises or team sports not only benefits physical health but also provides a powerful sense of camaraderie. The collective energy and shared experiences of these activities has the potential to uplift your spirits and reinforce your connection to others. Similarly, attending community events and workshops offers opportunities to learn and grow in a supportive environment. These activities encourage engagement and interaction, creating a sense of belonging that can counteract feelings of isolation.

While social connections are vital, it's equally important to strike a balance between community time and personal space. Regular social gatherings can be invigorating, yet it's essential to also allocate time for solitude and reflection. These quiet times are precious moments to recharge and process thoughts, ensuring that we remain grounded and centered. Scheduling regular social activities alongside moments of solitude can help maintain this balance. You can create a rhythm that includes both connection and introspection, cultivating a harmonious lifestyle that nurtures both your social and personal needs.

Decluttering for a Clear Mind

Cluttered spaces are a common source of stress for many people. A disorganized environment filled with scattered items and mess can heighten stress levels, making it difficult to focus or relax and increasing cortisol levels in the process. The psychological impact of clutter is notable, often contributing to feelings of anxiety and depression and leaving us feeling trapped in our own homes. In contrast, an organized living space promotes a sense of calm and control. A tidy environment improves our surroundings while positively impacting our mental state, helping us feel more at ease and think more clearly.

Embarking on a decluttering mission might feel daunting, but breaking it down into manageable steps can make the process more approachable. You can start by sorting your belongings into three categories: keep, donate, and discard. Be honest with yourself about what you truly need and what holds genuine value. Once you've categorized your items, organize your spaces by functionality. Designate specific areas for different activities, ensuring that everything has a place, and everything is in its place. This will make your home more efficient and more pleasant to be in. As you progress, you'll likely find that letting go of physical items brings unexpected emotional relief, as though you're shedding a layer of unnecessary weight.

Minimalism offers a framework for maintaining this newfound order. Rather than being about deprivation, it focuses on quality over quantity. Embracing a "less is more" mindset can reduce the clutter that weighs you down. This approach encourages us to invest in items that add true value to our life and to let go of those that don't. The liberation from material excess can lead to a more meaningful existence where joy comes from experiences and relationships rather than things. This shift in perspective can significantly reduce stress, as we're no longer surrounded by objects that demand our attention or resources.

Maintaining an uncluttered lifestyle requires ongoing effort, but simple habits can make it sustainable. Regularly review your possessions to assess their necessity, asking yourself if each item still serves a purpose or brings joy. Implementing a one-in-one-out rule for new purchases can also help keep your belongings in check. For every new item you bring into your home, let go of an old one. This practice encourages mindful consumption and prevents clutter from creeping back in.

So, remember: Decluttering is also a mental cleanse. As you clear your space, you clear your mind, making room for creativity, relaxation, and the things that truly matter. With less clutter, there will be more space for the life you want to build.

The Healing Power of the Outdoors

You step outside on a crisp morning, and the fresh air greets you like an old friend. Maybe you're heading to the park for a walk, or maybe you're just clutching a mug of tea on your balcony, staring into the distance like the main character in an indie film. Either way, you're doing something science enthusiastically approves of: engaging with nature. This isn't just a feel-good wellness trend; nature therapy, or ecotherapy, is a research-backed powerhouse for stress relief, hormone regulation, and keeping your cortisol levels from staging a hostile takeover.

We know that cortisol can wreak havoc on our body and mind if it's too high for too long, but perhaps we underestimate the effects that spending time outdoors can have on managing this hormone. A 20-minute walk in a green space has the potential to decrease cortisol levels by up to 21%, according to recent studies. Bonus points if you're near water or trees; these environments are particularly effective at calming the brain and reducing anxiety. Even seemingly mundane activities like walking your dog or gardening have a significant impact. Think about it: after a long day of adulting, doesn't it feel good to step away and hear actual birds chirping instead of email pings?

The calming effects of nature are supported by a wealth of scientific research. Exposure to natural environments has been linked to improved mood, reduced anxiety, and lower stress levels. Natural light regulates your body's internal clock, enhancing sleep quality. Fresh air invigorates the senses, helping to clear the mind

THE COMPLETE CORTISOL DETOX HANDBOOK

and improve focus. These elements work together to create an environment where the body can relax and rejuvenate, counteracting the stressors of everyday life. It's no surprise that time spent in nature is often described as restorative, offering a respite from the pressures of daily routines. Plus, there's something inherently satisfying about trading fluorescent lighting for sunlight and letting your mind wander without the pressure of productivity.

Engaging with nature doesn't have to be limited to traditional activities. There are countless creative ways to interact with the natural world. One interesting approach is through nature photography, capturing the beauty in the details of a flower or an expansive sunset. There's no need to have top-of-the-range tech equipment or artistic skills, as the aim is to encourage mindfulness. Simply focus on the present moment and appreciate the world around you. Sketching or painting outdoors can also be a fulfilling way to connect with nature, allowing your creativity to flourish in the open air. Organizing outdoor picnics with friends offers a social dimension to nature therapy, combining the benefits of community with the healing power of the outdoors.

Embrace the simple pleasures that the natural world has to offer. Take time to step outside, breathe deeply, and let the worries of each day dissolve into the background. Whether through a solitary walk or a shared experience with friends, these moments are precious and deeply restorative. So, the next time you're feeling overwhelmed, consider swapping screen time for green time. It might just be the easiest, most enjoyable health intervention you'll ever try.

Leisure and Creativity for Stress Relief

Finding space for leisure and creativity might seem like a luxury, yet these pursuits are vital for your mental health. Engaging in activities that spark joy and inspire creativity allows our mind to wander freely, providing a much-needed escape from stress.

Artistic expression, whether through painting, drawing, or any other medium, is a way to process emotions and explore new perspectives. When we immerse ourselves in creative tasks, we enter a state of flow where time seems to stand still, and worries fade into the background. This immersion provides immediate relief and cultivates a sense of accomplishment and fulfillment. Engaging in leisure activities like painting or drawing classes can rekindle your creative spirit, while writing poetry or journaling allows you to reflect and express yourself in ways that everyday conversations may not permit. These outlets encourage relaxation and provide a safe space to explore thoughts and feelings without judgment.

Play is not just for children; it holds significant benefits for adults as well. Incorporating play into your routine can inject a dose of fun and spontaneity into your life, improving your mood and reducing stress. Participating in board games with family can create bonds and laughter, providing a shared experience that strengthens relationships. Similarly, joining a recreational sports league can offer a physical outlet for stress relief while fostering a sense of teamwork and camaraderie. These playful activities remind us not to take life too seriously. They encourage us to enjoy the moment and embrace joy in its simplest forms.

With a busy schedule, it can be challenging to carve out time for leisure, but prioritizing these activities is another must. Whether it's a weekly art class or a quiet evening set aside for journaling, these dedicated times will allow you to fully engage in activities that nourish your soul. Protecting leisure time will most likely require setting boundaries and communicating clearly with others about your need for this time and space. However challenging this can be, it will create one more valuable safeguard against the pressures of daily life.

SEVEN
TACKLING THE HURDLES OF CORTISOL DETOX

LIFE IS BUSY—WE all know it. From juggling work deadlines to remembering to buy dog food before Max starts giving you the side-eye, it often feels like there's too much to do and not enough hours in the day. Managing time effectively involves so much more than crossing items off a to-do list. It's about using your energy and focus wisely to stay productive and, more importantly, sane. This is where tools like the Eisenhower Matrix come in handy.

Developed by Dwight D. Eisenhower—who, by the way, had to make slightly more pressing decisions than what's for dinner—the matrix helps sort tasks into four categories: urgent and important, important but not urgent, urgent but not important, and neither urgent nor important. It's a practical way to decide what truly needs your attention now versus what can wait, be delegated, or frankly ignored.

Research backs this structured approach to prioritization. Studies on cognitive load show that decision fatigue decreases productivity and increases stress. By having a clear framework like the matrix, you can reserve your mental energy for meaningful tasks, whether that's strategizing your next project at work, meal

TACKLING THE HURDLES OF CORTISOL DETOX

prepping for the week, or squeezing in a workout, all without feeling like the sky is falling. This framework will allow you to focus your energy where it matters most, aligning daily activities with your hormonal balance goals.

Creating a daily to-do list with focused priorities is an extension of this practice. Transferring thoughts to paper is an unburdening in itself, instantly decreasing mental load. This process is also very helpful when navigating a busy period, ensuring that efforts are directed toward high-priority tasks. If you're not accustomed to using organizational checklists, you can start by listing to-do items in the order of their importance and urgency, then tackle them systematically. This approach will prevent you from feeling overwhelmed and provides a sense of accomplishment as you check off each completed task. By keeping your to-do list concise, you will ensure that your focus remains sharp, allowing you to progress steadily toward your objectives.

Time-blocking techniques will bring another layer of structure to your day. Allocating specific blocks of time for hormone-balancing activities creates a dedicated space for nurturing your health. Schedule meal prep sessions to ensure you have nutritious options readily available, reducing the temptation to resort to less healthy choices when time is tight. Similarly, set aside time for exercise and mindfulness practices, treating them as essential appointments with yourself.

Distractions can easily derail even the most well-intentioned plans, making it crucial to develop strategies for maintaining focus. Implementing a no-phone policy during key tasks significantly enhances productivity. Create an environment free from digital interruptions to concentrate fully on the task at hand. Additionally, consider utilizing apps that block distracting websites, providing a virtual barrier against the lure of social media or online shopping. These tools empower us to reclaim our attention and channel it toward what truly matters.

Delegating tasks is another powerful strategy for managing

your time effectively. Enlist family members to help with chores, transforming household responsibilities into shared activities. This will lighten your load while building a sense of collaboration and unity within the household. For particularly demanding tasks, consider hiring assistance, whether it's a cleaning service or a meal delivery service. By sharing responsibilities, you will free up valuable time and energy, allowing you to focus on activities that support your health goals.

Time Management Challenge

Take a moment to pause and evaluate your daily tasks with this challenge. Use the Eisenhower Matrix to streamline your to-do list, reduce unnecessary stress, and optimize how you spend your time. Follow the steps below and write down your answers in a journal or planner. I also encourage you to reflect on the impact of this practice on your productivity and stress levels.

Step 1: Draw the Matrix

Create a simple four-quadrant grid labeled as follows:

- **Urgent & Important** (Top-left)
- **Not Urgent & Important** (Top-right)
- **Urgent & Not Important** (Bottom-left)
- **Not Urgent & Not Important** (Bottom-right)

Step 2: Brain Dump

SPEND 5 minutes listing all the tasks, appointments, and commitments currently on your mind. Don't worry about order—just get everything out.

Step 3: Categorize Your Tasks

Place each task from your list into the appropriate quadrant:

- **Quadrant 1**: Tasks that require immediate action (e.g., deadlines, emergencies).

- **Quadrant 2**: Tasks that require long-term planning (e.g., self-care, skill-building).
- **Quadrant 3**: Tasks you might be doing out of obligation but are not vital (e.g., interruptions).
- **Quadrant 4**: Tasks that are distractions or time-wasters.

Step 4: Take Action

- Focus your energy on **Quadrant 1** and **Quadrant 2** tasks.
- Delegate or minimize tasks in **Quadrant 3**.
- Eliminate tasks in **Quadrant 4** wherever possible.

Step 5: Reflect

Once you've completed your matrix, ask yourself:

- How can I prioritize my health and reduce stress by focusing more on Quadrant 2 tasks?
- Are there ways I can limit the number of urgent tasks to maintain better balance?

Pro Tips:

1. **Set Boundaries**: Learn to say no to non-essential tasks.
2. **Batch Tasks**: Group similar activities together to save time.

3. **Use Technology**: Try digital tools like Todoist or Notion to manage tasks.

Budget-Friendly Cortisol Detox

A TRIP to the farmer's market isn't just about picking up some kohlrabi and pretending you'll actually make a salad with it. It's an opportunity to make savvy, budget-friendly choices that actually support your body's hormonal health, without requiring fancy detox powders or overpriced juices. Seasonal produce, while often cheaper, is also packed with nutrients at their peak. Take summer strawberries, for example. Not only are they way tastier than their winter cousins, but they're also bursting with vitamin C and antioxidants, which is exactly what your body needs to tackle oxidative stress.

During a detox journey, these nutrients must be considered. They support the liver, bolster our immune system, and help keep energy levels stable (because let's face it, no one wants to be detoxing and hangry). Seasonal eating also means you're not stuck with bland options. Summer can be about fresh salads with ripe tomatoes and cucumbers, while fall might call for a warm roasted butternut squash. Why not save money while giving your body exactly what it needs? It's a win-win, without the need for extreme smoothies that taste like lawn clippings.

Another savvy shopping strategy is to utilize bulk buying for pantry staples. Think of items like grains, legumes, and nuts, which have a long shelf life and can be added to countless meals. Buying in bulk often reduces the price per unit, so you can stock up on ingredients that will support your detox efforts for weeks, if not months. This approach saves money and ensures you always have the building blocks for nutritious meals at hand, reducing the temptation to stray from your detox plan.

Community resources offer a wealth of opportunities to enhance your detox journey without a hefty price tag. Local fitness classes, often offered at community centers or parks, provide a sense of camaraderie and motivation. Participating in these classes will boost your physical health and create opportunities to build social connections, which are invaluable during any lifestyle change. Additionally, keep an eye out for free workshops or lectures on diet and health. These events can introduce you to new perspectives and tips, enriching your understanding of wellness in an engaging and interactive environment. Otherwise, if you are more inclined to exercise within the comfort of your own home, you can find an abundance of free quality workout videos online.

Managing finances effectively while on a hormonal reset plan doesn't have to feel restrictive. Start by creating a weekly meal plan. This simple act helps reduce food waste and ensures your diet aligns with your detox goals. By planning your meals, you can make the most of what you already have, minimizing unnecessary purchases. Setting a monthly wellness budget will allow you to allocate funds wisely, prioritizing the essentials that support your health without stretching your finances thin. This budget can include everything from groceries to occasional splurges on health classes or workshops.

Smart budgeting during a detox is really about making informed choices and embracing creativity. It's about finding joy in the simplicity of fresh, wholesome foods and the satisfaction of a life enhanced by mindful practices. So, before you drop half your paycheck on the latest detox trend that promises to fix everything from cortisol to caffeine addiction, consider heading to the market instead. Your body (and wallet) will thank you.

Personalizing Your Plan

DETOX PLANS AREN'T one-size-fits-all and, if they were, they'd probably fit about as well as those jeans I swore would stretch but never did. Bottom line is, your body is unique, and so are its needs. Effective detoxification depends on personalization, rooted in how your body responds to dietary changes, your specific health conditions, and even your lifestyle. For example, someone with lactose intolerance won't benefit from a detox smoothie loaded with whey protein, just as another with a packed schedule might struggle with an elaborate juice-cleanse regimen.

Our microbiomes, metabolic rates, and genetic predispositions all influence how we process nutrients and toxins. Tailoring your cortisol reset plan to fit your preferences and health history, whether that means focusing on liver-supportive foods like cruciferous vegetables or swapping out sugary drinks for hydrating herbal teas, makes the process more enjoyable and, crucially, sustainable. When your detox strategies align with your lifestyle, it's less of a punishment and more of a manageable, even rewarding, choice. So, ditch the generic plans and create one that works for you, because you deserve something that fits just right.

To begin crafting a plan that suits you, start by conducting a personal health inventory. Assess your current health status, identify any recurring challenges, and recognize what has or hasn't worked for you in the past. Reflect on your lifestyle, including stress levels, sleep patterns, and dietary habits, to gain a comprehensive understanding of your starting point. Once you have a clear picture, set realistic and attainable goals that align with your overall health objectives. These goals should be specific and measurable, allowing you to track your progress and celebrate achievements along the way. Remember, your goals should motivate you, not overwhelm you, so ensure they are within reach yet provide enough challenge to inspire growth.

Customizing your detox plan can be greatly enhanced by the use of digital tools. Apps designed for tracking dietary intake, exercise routines, and even meditation sessions can provide valuable insights into your habits and progress. They offer a convenient way to monitor your journey, providing reminders and encouragement as you move forward. Additionally, consulting with a nutritionist or wellness coach can lead to personalized advice tailored to your unique needs. These professionals can offer guidance on dietary adjustments, suggest supplements if necessary, and help you navigate any roadblocks that arise. Their expertise can be invaluable in ensuring your detox plan is both effective and safe.

Flexibility and adaptability are also essential components of a personalized detox plan. As you progress, regularly evaluate your plan to see what is working and what might need adjusting. Be open to making changes based on feedback from your body and results you observe. If a particular food isn't agreeing with you, find an alternative that provides similar benefits. If an exercise routine feels more draining than energizing, explore other activities that might suit you better. This willingness to adapt will ensure that your detox plan remains aligned with your evolving needs and goals.

Staying Motivated: Tips for Long-Term Success

ESTABLISHING WELL-DEFINED goals is fundamental to keeping up your drive during your detox journey. When goals are specific and measurable, they serve as a clear guide to success, allowing you to track progress and adjust as needed. The SMART criteria—Specific, Measurable, Attainable, Realistic, and Time-bound—offers a structured approach to goal setting. By defining what you want to achieve, whether it's increasing your daily vegetable intake or reducing caffeine consumption, you will create tangible targets to work toward.

To keep enthusiasm alive, it's important to celebrate the small milestones along the way. Each step forward is a victory, and acknowledging these achievements boosts morale and confidence. Create a reward system for yourself, where each milestone achieved is met with a personal treat, such as a new book or a relaxing day out. Visualizing success and its benefits also has an impact on maintaining motivation. Take a few moments each day to picture how achieving your goals will feel, the sense of pride and well-being that will accompany your progress. This mental imagery will reinforce your commitment and propel you forward, even on challenging days.

Accountability is another powerful motivator, providing an external source of encouragement and support. Forming a partnership with a detox buddy can make a significant difference, as you share experiences, challenges, and triumphs. This mutual support thrives through camaraderie and motivation, as you hold each other accountable and celebrate each other's successes. Additionally, participating in online forums or groups dedicated to detox and wellness can offer a broader support network. These communities provide a platform for sharing insights, asking questions, and receiving encouragement from like-minded individuals who understand the journey you're on. So, whether it's a partner, friend, or online group, having accountability measures in place helps maintain focus and reinforces your commitment to long-term success.

Motivation inevitably ebbs and flows, influenced by various factors. But by setting clear goals, celebrating milestones, drawing inspiration from others, and building a supportive network, you will have put in place a robust framework to sustain it. Remember that motivation is both the spark and the fuel, lighting the way toward a healthier you.

Handling Setbacks: Turning Challenges into Opportunities

MOST OF US have experienced the frustration of working toward a health goal, like sticking to a diet plan, only to have life throw a wrench into the mix. Maybe a work deadline derails your perfectly planned meals, or a friend's birthday dinner tempts you with your favorite dessert. These moments can feel like setbacks, but they are a normal part of any journey toward better health. Behavior change isn't linear. In fact, it is a process of trial, error, and adaptation.

Setbacks often help strengthen long-term habits by teaching us what doesn't work and why.

Instead of seeing these moments as failures, think of them as opportunities to fine-tune your approach. Didn't have time for meal prep? Stock your freezer with healthy, quick options for busy weeks. Faced with unexpected social temptations? Enjoy in moderation and balance it out later. Building resilience through these challenges is key to sustainable progress. Even the healthiest among us have their moments, because who hasn't had a "just one more slice" moment at a party? What really matters is how you regroup and keep moving forward.

Maintaining a positive mindset can make all the difference when navigating setbacks. Affirmations are a powerful tool in boosting confidence and reinforcing your commitment. Simple statements like "I am capable of overcoming challenges" can help shift your focus from the obstacle to your potential for success.

Try to embrace progress over perfection, recognizing that small steps forward are significant. Each day presents a new opportunity to learn and grow, and by focusing on your achievements rather than perceived shortcomings, you will cultivate a mindset of perseverance and positivity.

Life is beautifully messy and setbacks are as certain as the changing seasons. But just as each season brings its own beauty, each setback offers a chance to learn and grow. Teach yourself to embrace challenges, plan for disruptions, and develop a mindset of positivity to transform obstacles into opportunities for growth and strength.

CONCLUSION

Well, you've made it to the final chapter; cue the celebratory deep breath (or a well-earned sip of tea, wine, or whatever keeps you sane). By now, we've unpacked the science behind cortisol detox and how stress hormones can hijack everything from your sleep to your waistline to your ability to tolerate minor inconveniences. We've covered evidence-based strategies to bring your hormones back in balance, improve your sleep, and support your body's natural detox pathways. And if you've ever felt like stress was the uninvited guest running your life—whether it's the chaotic morning scramble, the never-ending to-do list, or those 3 a.m. reruns of every awkward thing you've ever said—this journey has been about taking back the reins.

Throughout this process, you've learned how daily practices like mindful breathing, regular movement, optimal sleep hygiene, and a nutrient-rich diet can lower stress levels and reset your body's natural rhythms. Whether it's swapping that third cup of coffee for green tea, prioritizing high-fiber foods for better gut health, or just taking a walk to clear your head, these small changes really do add up.

CONCLUSION

Now, as you stand at the threshold of what comes next, I encourage you to take action. Implement the strategies that resonate with you, share your experiences with others, and explore new aspects of wellness. Use this book as a springboard for your ongoing journey, a resource to revisit as you continue to evolve and grow. As a first step, it has not been a lesson on achieving perfection; instead, you have been learning to make choices that will help you feel better and function at your best. Remember, even those days when you accidentally eat the entire pint of ice cream or binge-watch a series until 2 a.m. aren't failures; they are opportunities for reflection, resets, and fresh starts. Your potential is limitless, and the power to shape your future lies within you.

Finally, I want to express my heartfelt gratitude to you, dear reader, for allowing this book to be a part of your life. I genuinely appreciate your trust and willingness to explore new paths of wellness and self-discovery. It is my hope that the insights and guidance provided have enriched your understanding and supported your journey toward better health.

As you close this book, take pride in the tools and knowledge you've gained, and keep experimenting with what works for you. After all, cortisol detox isn't a one-time fix, but a sustainable way to live healthier and feel more balanced.

Here's to your continued journey of enlightenment, strength, and flourishing well-being.

BONUS: TOP 30 CORTISOL DETOX RECIPES

Breakfast

<u>Superfood Chia Pudding with Berries and Almond Butter</u>

Ingredients

- 3 tablespoons chia seeds
- 1 cup unsweetened almond milk
- 1 teaspoon vanilla extract
- 1 teaspoon maple syrup (optional)
- 1/4 cup fresh berries (blueberries, raspberries, or strawberries)
- 1 tablespoon almond butter
- 1 tablespoon chopped almonds or granola (optional)

Procedure

1. Mix chia seeds, almond milk, vanilla extract, and maple syrup in a jar or bowl.
2. Stir well to prevent clumping, then refrigerate overnight (or at least 4 hours).
3. In the morning, top with fresh berries, almond butter, and chopped almonds or granola for added crunch.

Avocado and Egg Breakfast Bowl

Ingredients

- 1 ripe avocado, diced
- 2 large eggs, poached or boiled
- 1/4 cup cooked quinoa
- Handful of spinach or arugula
- 1 tablespoon olive oil
- Juice of 1/2 lemon
- Salt and pepper to taste

Procedure

1. Arrange spinach or arugula in a bowl and add quinoa, avocado, and eggs.
2. Drizzle with olive oil and lemon juice.
3. Sprinkle with salt and pepper, and serve immediately for a protein-packed start.

Adaptogenic Cacao Smoothie

Ingredients

- 1 frozen banana
- 1 cup unsweetened almond or oat milk
- 1 tablespoon raw cacao powder
- 1 teaspoon ashwagandha powder
- 1 tablespoon almond butter
- 1 teaspoon chia seeds
- 1/2 teaspoon cinnamon

Procedure

1. Blend all ingredients until smooth.
2. Pour into a glass and top with a sprinkle of cinnamon or cacao nibs.
3. Enjoy chilled as a stress-busting breakfast treat.

Savory Sweet Potato and Kale Hash

Ingredients

- 1 medium sweet potato, diced
- 1 cup chopped kale
- 2 eggs
- 1/4 teaspoon smoked paprika
- 1/4 teaspoon turmeric
- 1 tablespoon olive oil
- Salt and pepper to taste

Procedure

1. Heat olive oil in a skillet over medium heat. Add sweet potato, smoked paprika, turmeric, salt, and pepper. Sauté until tender (8–10 minutes).
2. Add kale and cook for an additional 2–3 minutes.
3. Push the veggies to one side and crack the eggs into the skillet. Cook to your preference.
4. Serve warm for a nutrient-rich, anti-inflammatory breakfast.

Gut-Healing Green Smoothie Bowl

Ingredients

- 1 frozen banana
- 1/2 cup frozen pineapple chunks
- 1 handful spinach or kale
- 1/2 avocado
- 1 cup unsweetened coconut water
- 1 teaspoon spirulina powder (optional)
- Toppings: sliced kiwi, chia seeds, shredded coconut, or granola

Procedure

1. Blend banana, pineapple, greens, avocado, coconut water, and spirulina until smooth.
2. Pour into a bowl and add toppings of your choice.
3. Serve immediately for a refreshing and energizing start to your day.

Turmeric Golden Oats with Toasted Walnuts

Ingredients

- 1/2 cup rolled oats
- 1 cup unsweetened almond milk or water
- 1/4 teaspoon ground turmeric
- 1/4 teaspoon cinnamon
- 1 teaspoon maple syrup or honey
- 1 tablespoon chopped toasted walnuts
- 1 tablespoon raisins or dried cranberries (optional)

Procedure

1. Cook oats in almond milk over medium heat, stirring frequently.
2. Add turmeric, cinnamon, and maple syrup, mixing well.
3. Once thickened, transfer to a bowl and top with walnuts, raisins, or other desired toppings.
4. Serve warm and enjoy the anti-inflammatory benefits.

Lunch

Salmon Buddha Bowl

Ingredients:

- 1 cup cooked quinoa
- 1 salmon fillet (grilled or baked)
- 1 cup steamed broccoli
- 1/2 avocado, sliced
- 1/4 cup shredded carrots
- 1 handful of mixed greens
- 2 tbsp sesame seeds
- 2 tbsp tamari or coconut aminos
- 1 tsp grated ginger
- 1 tsp sesame oil

Procedure:

1. Cook quinoa according to package instructions and set aside.
2. Grill or bake the salmon until flaky (about 12–15 minutes at 375°F).
3. Assemble the bowl by layering quinoa, broccoli, greens, carrots, and avocado.
4. Top with the salmon.
5. Mix tamari, ginger, and sesame oil into a dressing and drizzle over the bowl. Sprinkle with sesame seeds before serving.

Lentil and Spinach Curry

Ingredients:

- 1 cup cooked lentils
- 1 tbsp coconut oil
- 1/2 onion, diced
- 1 garlic clove, minced
- 1 tsp turmeric
- 1 tsp cumin
- 1/2 tsp paprika
- 1/2 tsp ground coriander
- 1 cup spinach leaves
- 1/2 cup canned coconut milk
- 1/2 cup diced tomatoes (fresh or canned)
- Fresh cilantro for garnish

Procedure:

1. Heat coconut oil in a pan and sauté onion and garlic until softened.
2. Add turmeric, cumin, paprika, and coriander. Cook for 1 minute.
3. Stir in tomatoes and coconut milk, then bring to a simmer.
4. Add lentils and spinach, cooking until spinach wilts (about 5 minutes).
5. Serve hot, garnished with fresh cilantro, alongside brown rice or quinoa.

Grilled Chicken and Avocado Wrap

Ingredients:

- 1 whole-grain tortilla
- 1 grilled chicken breast, sliced
- 1/4 avocado, mashed
- 1/2 cup mixed greens
- 1/4 cup shredded carrots
- 1 tbsp hummus
- Juice of 1/2 lemon

Procedure:

1. Spread mashed avocado and hummus over the tortilla.
2. Layer mixed greens, shredded carrots, and grilled chicken.
3. Squeeze fresh lemon juice on top, then roll tightly into a wrap.
4. Slice in half and serve with a side of fresh veggies or a small green salad.

Zucchini Noodle Stir-Fry with Tofu

Ingredients:

- 2 zucchinis, spiralized
- 1 block of firm tofu, cubed
- 1 tbsp olive oil
- 1/2 bell pepper, sliced
- 1/2 cup snap peas
- 1/4 cup tamari or coconut aminos

- 1 tsp minced ginger
- 1 tsp sesame oil
- 1 tsp honey (optional)

Procedure:

1. Heat olive oil in a skillet and sauté tofu until golden. Remove and set aside.
2. Add ginger, bell pepper, and snap peas to the skillet, cooking for 3–4 minutes.
3. Toss in zucchini noodles and cook for 2 minutes.
4. Return tofu to the skillet and add tamari, sesame oil, and honey (if using).
5. Stir well and serve warm.

Sweet Potato and Chickpea Salad

Ingredients:

- 1 medium sweet potato, roasted and diced
- 1 cup cooked chickpeas
- 2 cups arugula or spinach
- 1/4 cup pomegranate seeds
- 2 tbsp pumpkin seeds
- 2 tbsp olive oil
- Juice of 1 lemon
- 1 tsp ground cinnamon

Procedure:

1. Roast sweet potato cubes at 400°F for 25–30 minutes with a drizzle of olive oil and a sprinkle of cinnamon.

2. Toss arugula, chickpeas, roasted sweet potato, pomegranate seeds, and pumpkin seeds in a large bowl.
3. Drizzle with olive oil and lemon juice. Serve fresh.

Thai-Inspired Shrimp Lettuce Wraps

Ingredients:

- 1/2 pound cooked shrimp
- 1 head of butter lettuce (leaves separated)
- 1/2 cucumber, julienned
- 1/2 carrot, shredded
- 1/4 cup crushed peanuts (optional)
- 2 tbsp fish sauce or tamari
- 1 tbsp lime juice
- 1 tsp honey
- 1 tsp chili flakes (optional)

Procedure:

1. Mix fish sauce, lime juice, honey, and chili flakes in a small bowl for the dressing.
2. Layer shrimp, cucumber, and carrot onto each lettuce leaf.
3. Drizzle with dressing and sprinkle with crushed peanuts.
4. Fold the lettuce wraps and serve immediately.

Dinner

Turmeric Coconut Salmon with Quinoa

Ingredients:

- 4 salmon fillets
- 1 cup quinoa, rinsed
- 1 can (13.5 oz) coconut milk
- 1 tsp turmeric powder
- 1 tsp grated ginger
- 2 garlic cloves, minced
- 1 tbsp olive oil
- 1 cup spinach
- Salt and pepper to taste
- Fresh cilantro and lime wedges for garnish

Procedure:

1. Cook quinoa according to package instructions.
2. Heat olive oil in a skillet over medium heat. Add garlic and ginger, sauté until fragrant.
3. Stir in coconut milk, turmeric, salt, and pepper. Simmer for 5 minutes.
4. Add salmon fillets to the skillet, cover, and cook for 10 minutes or until salmon is cooked through.
5. Toss spinach into the skillet during the last 2 minutes of cooking.
6. Serve salmon and sauce over quinoa, garnished with cilantro and lime wedges.

Mediterranean Chickpea Bowl

Ingredients:

- 1 can chickpeas, rinsed and drained
- 1 cup cooked farro or brown rice
- 1 cucumber, diced
- 1 cup cherry tomatoes, halved
- 1/4 cup red onion, finely chopped
- 1/4 cup Kalamata olives
- 2 tbsp crumbled feta cheese
- 2 tbsp olive oil
- 1 tbsp lemon juice
- 1 tsp dried oregano
- Salt and pepper to taste

Procedure:

1. In a large bowl, combine chickpeas, farro, cucumber, tomatoes, red onion, olives, and feta.
2. Drizzle with olive oil and lemon juice.
3. Sprinkle oregano, salt, and pepper. Toss to combine.
4. Serve chilled or at room temperature.

Sweet Potato and Lentil Curry

Ingredients:

- 2 medium sweet potatoes, peeled and cubed
- 1 cup red lentils, rinsed
- 1 can (14 oz) diced tomatoes
- 1 can (13.5 oz) coconut milk

- 1 tbsp curry powder
- 1 tsp cumin powder
- 1 tsp turmeric powder
- 2 garlic cloves, minced
- 1 tbsp olive oil
- 2 cups vegetable broth
- Fresh cilantro for garnish

Procedure:

1. Heat olive oil in a large pot. Add garlic and spices, sauté for 1 minute.
2. Add sweet potatoes, lentils, tomatoes, coconut milk, and broth. Stir well.
3. Bring to a boil, then reduce heat to low. Simmer for 20-25 minutes, stirring occasionally, until sweet potatoes are tender.
4. Serve warm, garnished with fresh cilantro.

Zucchini Noodles with Avocado Pesto and Grilled Chicken

Ingredients:

- 2 medium zucchinis, spiralized
- 2 chicken breasts, grilled and sliced
- 1 ripe avocado
- 1/4 cup fresh basil leaves
- 2 tbsp pine nuts or walnuts
- 1 garlic clove
- 2 tbsp olive oil
- 1 tbsp lemon juice
- Salt and pepper to taste

Procedure:

1. Blend avocado, basil, nuts, garlic, olive oil, lemon juice, salt, and pepper into a creamy pesto.
2. Lightly sauté zucchini noodles in a pan for 2-3 minutes.
3. Toss noodles with pesto and top with grilled chicken slices.
4. Serve immediately.

Lemon Herb Baked Cod with Roasted Vegetables

Ingredients:

- 4 cod fillets
- 2 cups mixed vegetables (zucchini, bell peppers, carrots)
- 1 tbsp olive oil
- 1 tbsp lemon juice
- 1 tsp dried thyme
- 1 tsp dried rosemary
- 2 garlic cloves, minced
- Salt and pepper to taste

Procedure:

1. Preheat oven to 400°F (200°C).
2. Toss vegetables with olive oil, garlic, salt, and pepper. Spread on a baking sheet.
3. Place cod fillets on a separate baking sheet, drizzle with lemon juice, and sprinkle with thyme, rosemary, salt, and pepper.

4. Roast vegetables and cod in the oven for 15-20 minutes or until the fish flakes easily with a fork.
5. Serve cod with roasted vegetables on the side.

Quinoa-Stuffed Bell Peppers

Ingredients:

- 4 bell peppers, tops removed and seeds cleaned
- 1 cup cooked quinoa
- 1/2 cup black beans, rinsed and drained
- 1/2 cup corn (fresh or frozen)
- 1/2 cup diced tomatoes
- 1 tsp chili powder
- 1/2 tsp cumin powder
- 1/4 cup shredded cheese (optional)
- 1 tbsp olive oil
- Salt and pepper to taste

Procedure:

1. Preheat oven to 375°F (190°C).
2. In a bowl, mix quinoa, black beans, corn, tomatoes, chili powder, cumin, salt, and pepper.
3. Stuff the mixture into the bell peppers. Place in a baking dish.
4. Drizzle olive oil over the peppers. Cover with foil and bake for 30 minutes.
5. Remove foil, sprinkle with cheese if desired, and bake for another 10 minutes.
6. Serve warm.

Beverages

Adaptogenic Golden Milk Latte

A creamy, anti-inflammatory beverage to soothe stress and support hormonal balance.

Ingredients:

- 1 cup unsweetened almond or oat milk
- 1/2 tsp ground turmeric
- 1/4 tsp ground cinnamon
- 1/4 tsp ground ginger
- 1/2 tsp ashwagandha powder
- 1 tsp coconut oil
- 1 tsp raw honey or maple syrup (optional)
- Pinch of black pepper

Procedure:

1. Warm the almond or oat milk in a small saucepan over low heat.
2. Whisk in turmeric, cinnamon, ginger, ashwagandha, and black pepper.
3. Add coconut oil and continue stirring until well combined.
4. Remove from heat, sweeten with honey or maple syrup if desired, and serve warm.

BONUS: TOP 30 CORTISOL DETOX RECIPES

Berry-Ginger Stress Relief Smoothie

A nutrient-packed smoothie to stabilize blood sugar and fight oxidative stress.

Ingredients:

- 1 cup frozen mixed berries (blueberries, strawberries, raspberries)
- 1/2 banana
- 1/2 cup unsweetened Greek yogurt or plant-based yogurt
- 1 tsp freshly grated ginger
- 1 tbsp chia seeds
- 1 tsp maca powder
- 1/2 cup water or unsweetened almond milk

Procedure:

1. Blend all ingredients until smooth.
2. Pour into a glass and enjoy immediately.

Matcha Mint Refresher

An energizing, low-caffeine drink to enhance focus and reduce stress.

Ingredients:

- 1 tsp matcha powder
- 1/2 cup hot water (not boiling)
- 1/2 cup coconut water

- A few fresh mint leaves
- Juice of 1/2 lime
- 1 tsp raw honey (optional)

Procedure:

1. Whisk the matcha powder with hot water until frothy.
2. In a glass, combine coconut water, mint leaves, and lime juice.
3. Add the matcha mixture and stir. Sweeten with honey if desired.
4. Serve over ice.

Lavender Chamomile Lemonade

A calming beverage to relax the mind and body.

Ingredients:

- 2 cups water
- 2 chamomile tea bags
- 1 tsp dried culinary lavender
- Juice of 1 lemon
- 1-2 tsp raw honey or stevia (optional)
- Ice cubes

Procedure:

1. Boil the water and steep the chamomile tea bags and lavender for 5–7 minutes.
2. Strain the mixture and let it cool.
3. Add lemon juice and sweetener if desired.

4. Serve over ice.

Spiced Adaptogenic Hot Chocolate

A comforting treat with mood-boosting and stress-reducing properties.

Ingredients:

- 1 cup unsweetened almond milk
- 1 tbsp raw cacao powder
- 1/2 tsp cinnamon
- 1/4 tsp nutmeg
- 1/2 tsp reishi mushroom powder
- 1 tsp coconut sugar or raw honey (optional)
- Pinch of sea salt

Procedure:

1. Heat almond milk in a saucepan over low heat.
2. Whisk in cacao powder, cinnamon, nutmeg, reishi powder, and sea salt until smooth.
3. Sweeten with coconut sugar or honey if desired.
4. Pour into a mug and enjoy warm.

Green Detox Elixir

A refreshing juice loaded with antioxidants and detoxifying nutrients.

Ingredients:

- 1 cucumber
- 2 celery stalks
- 1 green apple
- 1 cup spinach
- Juice of 1/2 lemon
- 1-inch piece of fresh ginger
- 1/2 cup water

Procedure:

1. Blend all ingredients until smooth or use a juicer for a lighter texture.
2. Strain if desired, or enjoy it as is.
3. Serve chilled.

Desserts

Dark Chocolate Avocado Mousse

Rich in magnesium and healthy fats, this mousse promotes relaxation and reduces stress hormones.

Ingredients:

- 2 ripe avocados
- 1/3 cup unsweetened cocoa powder
- 1/4 cup maple syrup or honey
- 1/4 cup almond milk (or milk of choice)
- 1 tsp vanilla extract
- Pinch of sea salt

Procedure:

1. Scoop out the avocado flesh and place it in a blender or food processor.
2. Add cocoa powder, maple syrup, almond milk, vanilla extract, and sea salt.
3. Blend until smooth and creamy, scraping down the sides as needed.
4. Adjust sweetness or consistency with extra maple syrup or almond milk, if desired.
5. Serve in small bowls, and chill for 1 hour before enjoying.

Adaptogenic Hot Chocolate Energy Bites

Packed with adaptogens like ashwagandha, these bites offer stress-relieving benefits in a sweet package.

Ingredients:

- 1 cup dates (pitted)
- 1 cup raw almonds or walnuts
- 1/4 cup cacao powder
- 1 tsp ashwagandha powder
- 1 tsp cinnamon
- 1 tbsp coconut oil
- Pinch of sea salt

Procedure:

1. Soak dates in warm water for 10 minutes, then drain.
2. Blend nuts in a food processor until finely ground.
3. Add the remaining ingredients and blend until a sticky dough forms.
4. Roll into bite-sized balls and refrigerate for 1 hour before serving.

Berry Chia Pudding Parfait

Rich in omega-3s and antioxidants, this dessert helps reduce inflammation and stabilize blood sugar.

Ingredients:

- 1/4 cup chia seeds

- 1 cup unsweetened almond milk
- 1 tbsp maple syrup
- 1/2 tsp vanilla extract
- 1/2 cup mixed berries (blueberries, raspberries, strawberries)
- 1/4 cup granola (optional, for crunch)

Procedure:

1. Mix chia seeds, almond milk, maple syrup, and vanilla in a bowl. Let sit for 5 minutes, then stir to prevent clumping.
2. Refrigerate for at least 2 hours or overnight until thickened.
3. Layer chia pudding, berries, and granola in a glass or jar. Serve immediately.

Coconut Matcha Ice Cream

This dairy-free dessert combines matcha's calming properties with coconut's creamy texture.

Ingredients:

- 2 cups full-fat coconut milk
- 1/4 cup honey or maple syrup
- 1 tsp matcha powder
- 1 tsp vanilla extract

Procedure:

1. Blend all ingredients in a blender until smooth.

2. Pour the mixture into an ice cream maker and churn according to the manufacturer's instructions.
3. Freeze for an additional 1-2 hours for a firmer texture. Scoop and enjoy.

Banana Almond Butter Cookies

These naturally sweet cookies are high in potassium and protein, perfect for a stress-free snack.

Ingredients:

- 2 ripe bananas, mashed
- 1/2 cup almond butter
- 1 cup rolled oats
- 1 tsp cinnamon
- 1/4 cup dark chocolate chips (optional)

Procedure:

1. Preheat the oven to 350°F (175°C) and line a baking sheet with parchment paper.
2. Mix all ingredients in a bowl until well combined.
3. Drop spoonfuls of dough onto the baking sheet and flatten slightly.
4. Bake for 12-15 minutes until golden brown. Cool before serving.

Lavender Honey Yogurt Bark

A calming treat that combines lavender's soothing properties with probiotics for gut health.

Ingredients:

- 2 cups Greek yogurt
- 2 tbsp honey
- 1/2 tsp dried culinary lavender
- 1/4 cup sliced almonds
- 1/4 cup fresh blueberries

Procedure:

1. Mix Greek yogurt, honey, and lavender in a bowl.
2. Spread the mixture evenly on a parchment-lined baking sheet.
3. Sprinkle with almonds and blueberries.
4. Freeze for 2-3 hours or until firm. Break into pieces and store in the freezer until ready to eat.

POSTSCRIPT

First off, if you've made it to this page, congratulations—you stuck with me through *The Complete Cortisol Detox Handbook*! I hope this book has given you the tools, insights, and maybe even a few laughs to help you take control of your stress, balance your hormones, and feel like yourself again (instead of a caffeine-fueled, stress-ridden whirlwind).

Writing this book has been a labor of love, inspired by the incredible women I've worked with—women just like you—who are ready to stop letting stress run the show. My goal has always been to make science-backed wellness practical, doable, and maybe even a little enjoyable.

If you found this book helpful, I'd be truly grateful if you left a positive review on Amazon. Your feedback not only helps others find this book, but it also supports my mission to empower more people with the knowledge they need to feel their best.

Plus, good karma is real, and I hear it comes back around in the form of restful sleep and balanced hormones.

POSTSCRIPT

Wishing you health, balance, and many stress-free days ahead!

— *Sage O.*

THE EMERALD SOCIETY

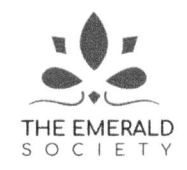

JOIN OUR TRIBE

The Complete Cortisol Detox Handbook

A Practical Guide & Workbook for Balancing Hormones, Regulating Emotions, Healing Your Gut, Reducing Inflammation and Managing Stress

A TES Publication © Copyright 2025 by Sage O'Reilley - All rights reserved

BIBLIOGRAPHY

- *Hormones – cortisol and corticosteroids* https://www.betterhealth.vic.gov.au/health/conditionsandtreatments/Hormones-cortisol-and-corticosteroids
- *Cortisol Levels during the Menopausal Transition and ...* https://pmc.ncbi.nlm.nih.gov/articles/PMC2749064/
- *Effectiveness of stress management interventions to ...* https://www.sciencedirect.com/science/article/pii/S0306453023003931
- *10 Natural Ways to Balance Your Hormones* https://www.healthline.com/nutrition/balance-hormones
- *Detox diets for toxin elimination and weight management* https://pubmed.ncbi.nlm.nih.gov/25522674/
- *ORGAN SYSTEMS: DETOXIfication* https://vetmed.tamu.edu/peer/detoxification/
- *Cortisol Detox: Effective Ways to Lower Stress Hormones* https://www.parsleyhealth.com/blog/cortisol-detox/
- *"Detoxes" and "Cleanses": What You Need To Know | NCCIH* https://www.nccih.nih.gov/health/detoxes-and-cleanses-what-you-need-to-know
- *11 Natural Ways to Lower Your Cortisol Levels* https://www.healthline.com/nutrition/ways-to-lower-cortisol
- *5-Day Hormone-Balancing Meal Plan* https://www.verywellfit.com/hormone-balancing-meal-plan-8304151
- *The effect of adaptogenic plants on stress: A systematic review ...* https://www.sciencedirect.com/science/article/pii/S1756464623002955#:~:text=Adaptogens%20might%20normalize%20chronically%20elevated,axis%20.
- *Stress, depression, diet, and the gut microbiota* https://pmc.ncbi.nlm.nih.gov/articles/PMC7213601/
- *Exercising to Relax - Harvard Health Publishing* https://www.health.harvard.edu/staying-healthy/exercising-to-relax
- *The Transformative Power of Yoga & Pilates for Mental ...* https://www.youngwellnessllc.com/the-transformative-power-of-yoga-and-pilates-for-mental-health
- *Exercise and stress: Get moving to manage stress* https://www.mayoclinic.org/healthy-lifestyle/stress-management/in-depth/exercise-and-stress/art-20044469

BIBLIOGRAPHY

- *How Strength Training Balances Your Hormones* https://experiencelife.lifetime.life/article/how-strength-training-balances-your-hormones/
- *Mindfulness from meditation associated with lower stress ...* https://www.ucdavis.edu/news/mindfulness-meditation-associated-lower-stress-hormone#:~:text=Individuals%20whose%20mindfulness%20score%20increased,resting%20cortisol%2C%22%20Jacobs%20said.
- *4-7-8 Breathing Technique* https://www.gundersenhealth.org/health-wellness/mental-health-relationships/4-7-8-breathing-technique
- *Empowering Women Through Mental Health: Strategies for ...* https://www.soulblissjourneys.com/post/empowering-women-through-mental-health-strategies-for-building-resilience
- *Technology and Stress: How to Take Control* https://www.itstimetologoff.com/2023/01/24/technology-and-stress-how-to-take-control/
- *The Impact of Sleep and Circadian Disturbance on ...* https://pmc.ncbi.nlm.nih.gov/articles/PMC4377487/
- *Women and Stress* https://my.clevelandclinic.org/health/articles/5545-women-and-stress
- *A Psychologist Shares 5 Benefits Of Making The 'Minimalist ...* https://www.forbes.com/sites/traversmark/2024/04/24/a-psychologist-shares-5-benefits-of-making-the-minimalist-switch/#:~:text=Competence.,experienced%20reduced%20anxiety%20and%20stress.
- *The effectiveness of nature-based therapy for community ...* https://www.nature.com/articles/s41598-023-49702-0
- *The Eisenhower Matrix: How to prioritize your to-do list* https://asana.com/resources/eisenhower-matrix
- *The 6 Best Budget-Friendly Anti-Inflammatory Foods ...* https://www.eatingwell.com/article/8024844/best-budget-friendly-anti-inflammatory-foods/
- *Be SMART about setting health-related goals | Aging* https://utswmed.org/medblog/smart-goals-health-wellness/
- *Healthy Communication Tips - Relationships* https://www.verywellmind.com/managing-conflict-in-relationships-communication-tips-3144967
- *Embracing Change: Transforming Your Life with Healthy ...* https://namigo.org/embracing-change-transforming-your-life-with-healthy-habits/
- *From Small Steps to Big Wins: The Importance of Celebrating* https://www.psychologytoday.com/us/blog/empower-your-

BIBLIOGRAPHY

- mind/202406/from-small-steps-to-big-wins-the-importance-of-celebrating
- *The Power of Storytelling - Anne McKeown* https://annemckeown.com/the-power-of storytelling/#:~:text=Story%20telling%20can%20provide%20healing%20and%20catharsis. Sharing%20personal%20experiences%2C%20whether%20joyful,trauma%20into%20resilience%20and%20growth.
- *Discovering Your Passions in Recovery: Building a Life You Love* https://www.newenglandrecoverycenter.org/blog/discovering-your-passions-in-recovery-building-a-life-you-love/#:~:text=A%20crucial%20part%20of%20this,reduce%20the%20risk%20of%20relapse.
- *cortisol — SUCCESS STORIES - Dr Arlo Gordin DC* https://www.drarlogordin.com/success-stories/tag/cortisol
- *Hormonal Imbalance: The Stress Effect | Kelsey-Seybold Clinic* https://www.kelsey-seybold.com/your-health-resources/blog/hormonal-imbalance-the-stress-effect#:~:text=Excess%20cortisol%20alone%20can%20contribute,these%20problems%20and%20adding%20others.
- *Mindfulness exercises* https://www.mayoclinic.org/healthy-lifestyle/consumer-health/in-depth/mindfulness-exercises/art-20046356
- *The top 10 empowering female communities online* https://www.reallywellness.co.uk/post/the-top-10-empowering-and-inspiring-female-communities-online
- *High Cortisol Levels the Stress Hormone Negative Effects* https://www.womenshealthnetwork.com/adrenal-fatigue-and-stress/negative-effects-of-high-cortisol/
- *How an Anti-inflammatory Diet Can Help Balance Hormones* https://naturalwomanhood.org/how-an-anti-inflammatory-diet-can-help-balance-hormones/
- *Somatic Exercises for Mental Health* https://www.charliehealth.com/post/somatic-exercises-for-mental-health
- *How To Reset The Adrenal System And Why It's Important* https://thrivenaturopathic.com/adrenal-gland-system-reset-detox/

Made in the USA
Monee, IL
19 April 2025